T0245134

Pig genetic resources in Europe

The EAAP series is published under the direction of Dr. P. Rafai

EAAP

EU

The European Association for Animal Production wishes to express its appreciation to the *Ministero per le Politiche Agricole e Forestali* and the *Associazione Italiana Allevatori* for their valuable support of its activities

Pig genetic resources in Europe

Characterisation and conservation

EAAP publication No. 104

Editors

L. Ollivier, F. Labroue, P. Glodek, G. Gandini and J.V. Delgado

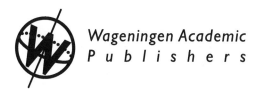

Wageningen Academic
P u b l i s h e r s

CIP-data Koninklijke
Bibliotheek, Den Haag

ISBN 9074134939 paperback
ISSN 0071-2477
NUGI 835

Subject headings:
Pig
Conservation
Genetic resources

First published, 2001

© **Wageningen Pers, Wageningen**
The Netherlands, 2001

CONTENTS

FOREWORD

Pig is a major source of protein for human populations. According to the FAO statistics of 1998, it accounts for about 38% of the world production of meat. Variations across continents however are important, since the pig contribution ranges from about 10% of the meat production in Africa to 53% in Asia. Europe is also a major area of pig production and consumption, since, for instance, pig meat has been representing about half of the meat consumed in the 15 countries of the European Union (EU) for the last ten years.

It is also well known that Europe as a whole shares a large part of the world pig genetic diversity, since nearly 46% of the breeds registered in the world inventory of FAO are found in Europe. The necessity to maintain this diversity and to develop alternative stocks for meeting a wide variety of production and market conditions is recognised, as well as the ensuing need to establish sound conservation programmes.

This book presents an overview of the situation of the pig genetic resources in four major pig producing countries of EU, namely France, Germany, Italy and Spain. The work carried out since 1996 in the evaluation of those resources and in their conservation has received support from the European Commission (EC) under the contract CEE RESGEN-CT95-012, in short RESGEN12, entitled *"European gene banking project for pig genetic resources"*. This support has been granted in the general context of the RESGEN programme, launched by the EU Directorate-General for Agriculture as an implementation of the EC regulation 1467-94 on *"the conservation, characterisation, collection and utilisation of genetic resources in agriculture"*.

The book is divided up into four sections, each of which corresponds to one of the specific objectives and tasks identified in the RESGEN12 project. Section I addresses the *primary characterisation* of the breeds included in the project. It presents general information and so-called "passport data", such as data available in various national or international databases. This section also includes information on pedigrees whenever such data are recorded. Section II on *performances* presents additional information on reproduction and production performances, as well as any specific qualification of each breed. Section III on *genetic distances* is devoted to within and between-breed genetic variability evaluated through various genetic markers, exhibiting immunological, biochemical or DNA polymorphisms. Finally, section IV on *semen collections* provides details on the *ex situ* conservation programmes operated in the four countries and it presents the status of the collected germplasm at the end of the project.

The emphasis is on local breeds, most of them maintained in specific production systems and linked to regional policies stressing product quality and environment integration. The book is therefore completed by a map of Europe showing the regional coverage of the 23 pig breeds considered in the project, and photographs of animals representative of each of these breeds.

The information gathered is intended as a basis for rationalising the conservation of European pig genetic resources, through a comprehensive evaluation of the breeds performances and qualifications, as well as of their diversity at the gene level. Conservation policies are outlined, addressing both live animals and cryopreserved germplasm. In particular, recommendations are given for establishing gene banks for local breeds exposed to serious risks of genetic erosion, if not complete extinction. In this context, an evaluation is made of the cryopreservation techniques presently available for establishing pig gene banks and potential developments allowed by the most recent progress in reproductive technologies in the pig are also discussed.

In the 12 chapters of the book, contributions from a number of European experts in the field of pig production and genetics, conservation genetics and reproductive physiology are put together. The book should thus be of interest to a wide audience throughout the pig industry. Students and researchers will also find in it information of scientific interest on a very diverse sample of breeds. And finally, the economic dimension given to the various conservation strategies should be of benefit to decision-makers in the area of domestic animal conservation under European conditions.

This book is the result of a variety of national and international efforts. The editors wish to express their gratitude for the support of the European Commission throughout the work carried on during the last 5 years. In addition to the RESGEN12 contract mentioned above, the support provided for evaluating genetic diversity (EC Framework IV programme: contract BIO4-CT98-0188 on *"Characterisation of genetic variation in the European pig to facilitate the maintenance and exploitation of biodiversity"*) is also gratefully acknowledged. Collection of country information on pig breeds relies on the European National Co-ordinators within the FAO Global Strategy for the Management of Farm Animal Genetic Resources and they should all be thanked for their contributions to the breeds' characterisation. Additional support has been provided by the French Ministry of Agriculture and "Bureau des Ressources Génétiques" in Paris. Special thanks are also due to F. Bariteau, M. Molénat (INRA) and C. Tixier (ITP) for their actions in the conservation of French local breeds. The Italian programme has received support from ELPZOO and special thanks are due to O. Franci (University of Florence), G. Madonia (ISZ, Palermo) and D. Matassino (ConSDABI, Benevento). The Italian programme has received additional financial support from ELPZOO Foundation, the National Research Council and the "Istituto Sperimentale Zootecnico", Palermo. Thanks are due to A.N.A.S, ConSDABI, MiPA Gestione ex ASFD (Siena), APA (Siena) and S.O.A.T. Regione Sicilia for their work in conservation of Italian local pig breeds. And, finally, the editorial support of the staff at INRA "Station de Génétique Quantitative et Appliquée" (Jouy-en-Josas), particularly Marie-Laure Le Paih, Françoise Bouchain, Hervé Lagant and Sylvie Nugier, is also gratefully acknowledged.

It is hoped that the results presented in this book will help in the management and conservation of pig genetic resources over the whole European continent and in other countries of the world as well. May the book also stimulate further work for extending our knowledge of the pig and other farm animal species genetic diversity, and so help in building more efficient strategies for the maintenance and sustainable use of biodiversity.

The Editors
L. Ollivier, F. Labroue, P. Glodek, G. Gandini and J.V. Delgado

SECTION I

INVENTORY OF THE PIG GENETIC RESOURCES IN EUROPE (PRIMARY CHARACTERISATION)

Chapter 1.1. An overview of the genetic resources of pigs and their management and conservation

L. Ollivier[1], J. Wrede[2] and O. Distl[2]

[1]*INRA-Station de Génétique Quantitative et Appliquée, 78350 Jouy-en-Josas, France*
[2]*School of Veterinary Medicine, Bünteweg 17p, 30559 Hannover, Germany*

1. Introduction

The pig is a major source of protein for human populations. According to the FAO statistics it accounts for about 38 % of the world production of meat. Regional variations however are important, as pig meat only represents 10 % of the total meat production in Africa, whereas in China this percentage reaches 85 %. Europe is a major area of production since, for instance, pig meat is representing about half of the meat consumption in the 15 countries of the European Union (EU).

The pig is mainly fed on grain, which developed countries tend to overproduce, while developing countries are badly in need of such food resources. Man and pig compete for food and the management of pig genetic resources should be envisaged in the perspective of the most efficient use of whatever feed resources are available (Epstein and Bichard, 1984). Various aspects of domestication, the present use of pig breeds and their conservation have already been dealt with in several reports, such as those by Epstein and Bichard (1984), Molénat and Legault (1986), Jonsson (1991), King (1991) and Steane (1991).

This chapter is partly based on an FAO Animal Production and Health paper on *The management of global animal genetic resources* (see Ollivier and Molénat, 1992). We shall here review the objectives assigned to the management of the pig genetic resources, the situation of those resources in various regions of the world, and the identification of priority breeds which deserve preservation/development action. The emphasis is on indigenous breeds in 3 continents, namely Asia, Latin America and tropical Africa, as a basis for putting the European pig genetic resources in a proper global perspective.

2. Management of genetic resources in pigs: general considerations

Potential resources include a wide spectrum of pig populations, which may be classified, according to a typology suggested by Lauvergne (1982), into four categories by increasing degree of evolution: (1) wild (or feral) populations, (2) traditional (or indigenous) populations, (3) standard breeds, and (4) selected lines (and so-called "new breeds"). Though a somewhat different classification has been retained by Mason (1988) in his dictionary, one can easily find in this compilation of over 500 pig breeds listed, representatives of all four categories of populations, with a marked predominance of categories (2) and (3).

Management of genetic resources is usually understood in a longer term perspective than is the case for current breeding schemes oriented towards meeting rather short/medium term requirements. The goal is, in a long-term perspective, to maintain genetic variability, be it quantitative or qualitative (Ollivier and Lauvergne, 1988). In pigs, like in other livestock species, there is at present no indication that genetic variability is at risk for the traits usually considered by farmers and given present conditions of breeding (Fredeen, 1984). The highly polygenic nature of such traits, combined with systems of matings which largely favour outbreeding, are expected to prevent against any significant decay of genetic variability. In addition, between-breed variation is generally thought to be the result of different frequencies of genes shared in common by several populations rather than of presence/absence of individual genes. In contrast, the risk of loss of variability may be greater for qualitative variation, especially when it has a monogenic basis. The difficulty here is that our genetic knowledge of pig populations is presently too limited to allow tracing the population-gene combinations really at risk with sufficient accuracy.

Another, and perhaps more important, concept underlying genetic resources is genetic flexibility. Even assuming that the genetic variability available makes possible, in theory, changes in any population in any direction for any trait, flexibility in pig evolution is somewhat constrained by the multiplicity of objectives to be considered. Each one of these objectives needs an appropriate allocation of the limited opportunities for selection and is also constrained by the differing amounts of genetic variability depending on the trait considered. Between breeds diversity plays an essential role by allowing changes to be made rather quickly to cope with new situations. An example is the repopulation of Haiti after the outbreak of African swine fever in 1983. The use of a combination of the *Créole* pig from a neighbouring island (Guadeloupe), a local European breed (*Gascon* from France) and the highly prolific Chinese breeds (*Taihu*) quickly provided genotypes well adapted to the variable and generally extremely harsh rural environment (Delatte *et al.,* 1991). Because of their low heritability, traits related to fitness, such as fertility, longevity, general disease resistance, are particularly valuable criteria for deciding on priorities for conservation/development action.

Our limited knowledge of several aspects of the pig's biology calls for further scientific investigations and some extreme genotypes may be of great utility for that purpose. Such is the case, for instance, with the European Wild Pig and the Chinese *Meishan* in the European pig gene mapping project (Archibald, 1997). A final point in this regard is the preservation of a world heritage, though in this respect the pig has a much less fashionable image in most of our societies than other farm animals.

A proper assessment of the available resources is of fundamental importance. Breeds have to be catalogued and evaluated. Information on pig breeds can be found in scientific literature and, more recently, following European and Asian initiatives, regional and global data banks have been established. The catalogue by Mason (1988) provided an early overview of the distribution of pig breeds across the world. As shown in table 1, nearly 400 breeds were then registered as being currently exploited, the largest numbers of breeds being found in Asia and Europe. More detailed information can be found in several data banks, such as the EAAP Global Animal Genetic Data Bank established in 1986 (Simon and Buchenauer, 1993) and the FAO Domestic Animal Diversity Information System (DAD-IS) launched in 1996 (see Appendix for web addresses). Since then, the world breeds information has been updated at FAO) on a regular basis and the most recent situation has been published by Scherf (2000). Table 2 shows for pigs a marked overall increase in the number of breeds registered, as well as in the proportion of breeds endangered.

Table 1. An overview of pig breeds, types and varieties across the world (from Mason, 1988).

Breed	Africa	America	Asia and Oceania	Europe	Total
Important	1	11	15	4	71
Secondary	6	40	134	77	257
Rare	-	5	3	39	47
Extinct	-	16	9	114	139
Total	7	72	161	274	514

Table 2. The present world situation of pig breeds and their risk status (from Scherf, 2000).

Breed risk status	Number of breeds[1]				
	Africa	America	Asia and Oceania	Europe	Total
Unknown	6	27	60	18	111
Not at risk	12	14	109	88	223
Endangered[2]	2	8	12	84	106
Critical[2]	2	13	5	38	58
Extinct	1	31	14	105	151
Total	23	93	200	333	649

[1]Breeds are defined as country populations, and include commercial lines. Same breeds may be present in different countries.
[2]Endangered (Critical) risk status is defined by FAO as corresponding to less than 1000 (100) breeding females or 20 (5) breeding males.

In practice, genetic resources are managed using classical breeding plans, implying evaluation of either individual breeding values (for pure breeding) or of population mean values (for crossbreeding schemes), as reviewed by Glodek (1991). For conservation, live populations and cryoconservation can be used, as in other farm species. A.I. and the use of frozen semen have an important role to play (see chapters 4.1 and 4.2 of this book).

At world level, a new impetus has been given to the management of genetic resources in the early 1990s, particularly by the Convention on Biological Diversity of 1992. A Global Strategy for the Management of Farm Animal Genetic Resources has been recommended by FAO and is now operational. This Strategy covers activities such as the monitoring of existing animal genetic resources, *in situ* and *ex situ* conservation programmes, training and communication. The whole programme relies upon a geographically distributed structure implying national and regional co-ordination (see Scherf, 2000).

3. Regional survey outside Europe

3.1. Asia

More than half of the world pig population is located in Asia, with an inventory of around 520 million heads. China represents the most of it with about 420 million, followed by Vietnam with 15 million. The enormous Chinese reservoir of genetic diversity for pigs, among other farm animals, was first drawn to the world's attention by Epstein (1969) and later documented by Legault (1978) and Cheng (1984). In addition to results collected in China, research findings on a few local Chinese breeds imported by several western countries are also available.

China has a long history of domestication, going back more than a hundred centuries (Zhao, 1990). It is therefore likely that domestication in China started not later than and independently of the domestication centre of Near-East Asia. A long tradition of pig husbandry under various climatic and geographic conditions is probably a major cause of the presently observed genetic diversity. From reports based on a comprehensive investigation launched in 1981 by the Chinese government (Zhang, 1986), the number of native breeds officially registered was about 50, to which 25 improved breeds (including imported foreign breeds) should be added. The local breeds belong to 6 different types: North China, Central China, Shanghai area, South China, Southwest China and Plateau. The more complete FAO inventory now includes 118 breeds.

Phenotypic variability among breeds is extremely large. In an attempt to characterise Chinese breeds by their phenotypic traits, Li and Enfield (1989) were able to classify 75 breeds into 6 clusters, mainly based on litter size and body weights. As shown in table 3, the range between extreme type averages was about 8 piglets for litter size (from 6.4 to 14.5) and over 200 kg for adult body weight (from 33 to 242 kg).

Table 3. Characterisation of Chinese breeds of pigs (from a cluster analysis by Li and Enfield, 1989).

	Characteristics		Type average		Breed example	
Type	Prolificacy	Size at birth	Piglet/litter	Adult body weight (kg)	Name	Origin
I	medium	small	9.9	91	*Hainan*	South
II	medium	medium	10.8	165	*Beijing Black*	New
III	medium	large	10.4	242	*Yorkshire*	Foreign
IV	high	medium	14.5	151	*Meishan*	Shanghai
V	high	small	13.4	116	*Jinhua*	Central
VI	low	very small	6.4	33	*Tibetan*	Plateau

Among Chinese breeds, the *Taihu* group certainly deserves priority attention, because of the high prolificacy (going along with corresponding maternal abilities such as teat number) and the early sexual maturity of those breeds. Their merit under Chinese production conditions has been confirmed under intensive husbandry conditions in several other countries: see Legault and Caritez (1983) for one of the earliest evaluation of the *Meishan* and *Jiaxing* breeds outside China. According to King (1992), the *Taihu* group in the early 1990s included seven genetically distinct breeds, some of them divided into strains (*e.g. Meishan*). the group had an estimated 600 000 breeding animals, with a tendency to an increase in popularity of the *Erhualian* breed. None of those breeds was really in danger of extinction. Breeding was well organized and structured, and a clear hierarchy of herds existed. The danger for the future was seen as coming from an increased consumer demand for lean meat, which would put pressure on crossing with exotic breeds and expose *Taihu* breeds to the risk of genetic dilution of their favourable reproductive characteristics. Importation of foreign stock has indeed been increasing over the last 10 years, with an increase in crossbreeding and a concomitant decrease in the demand for purebred females. Conservation herds for both *Meishan* and *Erhualian* have therefore been established in several state farms (C. Legault, 2000, personal communication).

Opportunities for meeting other requirements are also reported in Chinese breeds, such as resistance to extreme cold weather in the *Min* breed of North China, which appears to combine this favourable trait with high prolificacy. Special food-seeking abilities are mentioned for the Tibetan pig, which combines dwarfism with adaptation to cold, alertness and highly developed digestive organs able to utilize shrubs, stems, roots and seeds of wild plants.

Vietnam, the second largest pig producing country in Asia, relies on both intensive production systems and household production, the latter however representing 80 % of the total output. Vietnam also shares with South-East Asia some unique features in the role played by the pig: fat as a source of essential fatty acids, manure as fertilizer for rice cultivation and frequent association with fish production. Vietnam has an abundance of local breeds, several extremely early reproducing, among which the *Mong Cai* is considered as a genetic type of interest for the future and currently under investigation in several state farms (Molénat and Tran The Thong, 1991).

3.2. Latin America and Caribbean zone

Indigenous pigs of this region actually derive from early importations. According to Epstein and Bichard (1984), pigs were introduced from China in the 15th century, and the colonists in the 16th century brought along both Celtic and Iberian types. To-day indigenous breeds play a role depending on the production system. Beside intensive production based exclusively on improved breeds such as *Large White*, *Landrace* or *Duroc*, Latin America has an important sector of small-holder production, with moderate productivity and low inputs, which relies on local breeds either pure or used in crosses with improved breeds. Backyard pigs raised for self-consumption are also a constant feature of meat production in that region of the world and Criollo types usually serve that purpose: see chapter 1.2 for the *Créole* pig of Guadeloupe.

Half of the pigs of that region live in Brazil. In 1986, a project for evaluating national breeds of pigs was started in South Brazil (Primo, 1987) under the auspices of the Agricultural Research Corporation (EMBRAPA) and of the National Centre for Genetic Resources (CENARGEN). State support is provided for four breeds, *Moura*, *Caruncho*, *Pirapitinga* and *Piau*, and conservation nuclei for the latter breed have been established in the 3 southern provinces of Brazil. Crossbreeding experiments with improved breeds are carried on in the Santa Catarina and Parana provinces. The objective is to obtain more precise information on the specific characteristics of those rather numerous local breeds, their nutritional requirements, their ability to survive in harsh environmental conditions and their possible resistances to diseases (Mariante, 1990).

Mexico also has several local breeds of interest, generally of small size and well adapted to various climates. The black hairless pig of Yucatan, in addition to being a natural miniature pig of about the same size as other artificially created strains (Panepinto *et al.*, 1978), is reportedly well adapted to hot climates and to bulky diets. The *Cuino* miniature pig (10-12 kg adult weight), though nearly extinct according to Mason (1988) and Scherf (2000), would deserve being conserved, as it is reported to be able to survive long periods of starvation under household conditions.

3.3. Tropical Africa

The pig population of tropical Africa is about 7.3 million, half of which is located in the coastal region of West Africa, from Senegal to Cameroon. The West African indigenous pig belongs to the Iberian type and includes such varieties as the *Ashanti* dwarf in Ghana, the *Bakosi* in Cameroon and the Nigerian native (Mason, 1988). This pig may have migrated from Northern Africa and Egypt (Pathiraja and Oyedipe, 1990), or, according to Epstein (1971), it could derive from early Portuguese imports in lower latitudes.

This type of pig is well adapted to the extensive conditions of the traditional village management, since it gets its food essentially from scavenging. It constitutes a valuable source of meat for the small-scale farmers of that region. In more intensively cultivated areas, indigenous pigs are kept under semi-intensive systems and fed agricultural by-products.

West African pigs grow slowly, produce small litters, partly because of an excessively early sexual precocity with a first farrowing at 8 month of age, but sows reproduce with regularity and may farrow 2.3 litters a year (Pathiraja and Oyedipe, 1990). There are indications that indigenous pigs may exhibit better heat and parasite tolerance than exotic breeds, and also better disease tolerance and trypanotolerance. However, these are field observations which would require the support of experimental evidence.

The best described genetic situation is that of the Nigerian native by Pathiraja and Oyedipe (1990). Between 1975 and 1985, a steady decline of the percentage of indigenous pigs has been observed, from 89 percent of the total in 1975 to 58 percent in 1985. As a consequence, in several major pig producing areas, indigenous pigs are virtually extinct. The same authors point to a possible contribution of inbreeding to the low productivity observed under traditional management systems, owing to the small size of individual herds.

In addition to Nigeria, where scientific investigations on native and crosses with exotic breeds have been carried on, work done in Zimbabwe (Pig Industry Board) and in Benin should also be mentioned. As pig is a species of relatively minor importance in Africa, the lack of accurate statistics and basic production data, recognized as a major constraint for an adequate management of farm animal genetic resources in this part of the world (Setshwaelo, 1990), applies even more to African indigenous breeds of pigs.

3.4. Other regions

Local breeds of pigs in other parts of the world outside Europe will be briefly mentioned here for the sake of completeness. The conservation of rare breeds has received considerable attention in recent years as well as support from various state and private institutions in Canada and U.S.A., through Rare Breed and Minor Breed Conservancy associations. In India, a National Bureau of Animal Genetic Resources has been established and is engaged in conservation and management of native populations, and studies on local breeds of pigs are reported from several research teams. Japan has implemented a comprehensive conservation programme aimed at examining native breeds as a possible source of genes for quality products (Scherf, 2000). Australia and New Zealand have no local breeds as they rely on imported British breeds, some of which have become feral since their introduction on this continent. Particular mention should be made of the village pig in the civilization of Papua-New-Guinea.

4. The European situation

Europe has a long history of animal selection which has resulted in a large number of breeds still existing in the major livestock species. Though Europe is the 2nd smallest continent it has the largest number of breeds for several major species (Scherf, 2000). This is also true for pigs, for which the European share in number of breeds (45.8 %) largely exceeds its share in number of heads (21.5 %).

A continuous effort of inventory and characterisation of breeds was launched in the early 1980s by the European Association for Animal Production (EAAP). This effort eventually led to the creation of an Animal Genetic Data Bank (EAAP-AGDB) at the School of Veterinary Medicine of Hanover in 1987 (for a detailed historical overview of European breed inventories see Ollivier, 1998). This section will essentially rely on the information available at EAAP-AGDB (see Appendix), excluding extinct breeds. Table 4 shows that the information available presently covers 185 breeds of pigs. Their status of endangerment is evaluated on the basis of effective population size, from which an expected increase in inbreeding over 50 years can be derived, assuming a generation interval of 1.5 years (as explained in Simon and Buchenauer, 1993). Additional factors of risk such as population trend, number of herds and percentage of purebreeding are also considered. It should however be emphasised that status of endangerment in table 4 is only defined for native breeds. On this basis, 33 breeds appear as being endangered, more or less severely, 28 of which are located within the European Union (EU). The comparison of these figures with the 122 European breeds considered at risk in the FAO inventory (see endangered + critical in table 2) illustrates the fact that risk status defined within country, on the sole basis of country population numbers as explained in table 2, may not reflect the status of the breeds regionally, as also noted by Scherf (2000).

Table 4. Pig breeds in the EU and their status of endangerment according to EAAP-AGDB.

Country	Number of breeds according to their status of endangerment							
	Unknown	Not defined[1]	Not endangered	Potentially endangered	Minimally endangered	Endangered	Critically endangered	Total
Austria	2	-	-	-	-	-	-	2
Belgium	-	1	2	-	-	-	-	3
Denmark	1	2	1	-	-	1	1	6
Finland	-	1	1	-	-	-	-	2
France	-	24	-	2	-	3	1	30
Germany	-	13	-	-	-	2	1	16
Ireland	-	3	-	-	-	-	-	3
Italy	2	5	-	-	1	-	4	12
Luxembourg	-	1	-	-	-	-	-	1
Netherlands	-	3	-	-	-	-	-	3
Portugal	-	-	-	1	-	-	1	2
Spain	3	-	3	-	-	-	7	13
Sweden	-	4	1	-	-	-	-	5
UK	-	5	6	3	-	-	-	14
Total EU	8	62	14	6	1	6	15	112
Rest of Europe	5	54	9	1	-	-	4	73
TOTAL	13	116	23	7	1	6	19	185

[1]for the purpose of this table, degree of endangerment is defined only for *native* breeds, *i.e.* breeds originating from the country.

The large number of non-native breeds, therefore with undefined status in table 4, deserves further explanations (see particularly the cases of France and Germany). One main reason is the inclusion of populations such as *selected lines* or *exotic breeds*, usually maintained either as commercial lines in breeding companies or for research purposes by state institutions. Another reason is the inclusion of country varieties of major international breeds, such as *Large White, Landrace, Piétrain*, and the American *Hampshire* and *Duroc*. Table 5 shows their distribution across the European continent. The survey of Sutherland *et al.* (1985) clearly indicated that breeds called *Large White* (or *Yorkshire*) and *Landrace* were present in most European countries before 1970. *Piétrain* was also represented before 1970 in one out of 3 countries surveyed, whereas *Hampshire* and *Duroc* were only present in 2 countries. The next decade was marked by extensive breed migrations, including importations of the latter two American breeds and also exchanges of *Landraces*, mostly of Scandinavian origin, among European countries.

The presence of those breeds in the EAAP-AGDB records largely reflects this past history, though a reduction in the total number of such breeds since 1981, from 106 to 72, is observed. This reduction is probably due to an incomplete recording, since not all countries include this category of breeds in their inventories. In several cases also, imported breeds served to develop commercial lines by breeding companies, either as pure or composite lines. In fact, referring again to the population typology mentioned earlier (in 2.), the international breeds of table 5 may be seen as being in transition from their traditional status of *standard breed* to the next domestication stage of *selected line*. Such lines are not either included in most country inventories.

Table 5. Major international breeds of pig: distribution of country varieties of the same breed across Europe.

Breed	Number of breed varieties present in the European countries				
	Before 1970[1]	Imported between 1970 and 1981[1]	In 1981[1]	In 1993[2]	In 2001[3]
Large White	26	-	26	17	20
Landrace[4]	24	14	38	22	24
Piétrain	8	1	9	4	5
Hampshire	2	14	16	6	11
Duroc	2	15	17	7	12
Total	62	44	106	56	72

[1]based on a survey of 25 European countries by Sutherland *et al.* (1985): situation of 1981.
[2]Simon and Buchenauer (1993).
[3]EAAP-AGDB.
[4]Belgian *Landrace* excluded.

The previous considerations on the variety of genetic resources which can be put under the general name of "breed" (or, more specifically, under the name of for instance *Large White* breed in a country) show the difficulty to properly assess the genetic resources of a region such as Europe and evaluate their vulnerability to genetic erosion. Obviously the concept of *breed similarities* across various countries, developed by Simon and Buchenauer (1993), has to be taken into account when establishing management/conservation plans.

One of the purposes of the EAAP-AGDB is the monitoring of current conservation activities. It is known that in pigs, like in the other species, the conservation of rare breeds has received considerable attention in Europe, implying support from government as well as from industry and private organisations, as detailed for instance by Ollivier *et al.* (1994). Conservation is mainly achieved *in situ* and completed by cryoconservation of frozen semen, using techniques which will be detailed in section IV of this book. The pig cryoconservation programmes registered in EAAP-AGDB are presented in table 6. It can be seen that such programmes are still very few in Europe, since only about half of the breeds in some danger of extinction can rely on stores of frozen semen, and most of these include less than 20 boars. It should however be noted that the situation reported in table 6 is that which prevailed before the launching of the RESGEN project.

Table 6. Pig cryoconservation programmes in Europe using frozen semen (number of breeds cryopreserved and number of boars sampled per breed).

	Breed status of endangerment			
	Not defined	Not endangered	Endangered	Total
Part of Europe				
European Union	-	2	10	12
Rest of Europe	1	1	-	2
Number of boars per breed				
5 or less (or unknown)	1	1	1	3
5-20	-	1	9	10
Above 20	-	1	-	1
Total number of breeds	1	3	10	14
Total number of boars	3	58	88	149

It can also be seen that conservation efforts appear in some cases to be directed towards genetic resources that are not really at any risk. This may therefore appear as misdirected spending decisions, because they were probably taken within national contexts. On the other hand, it may be argued that the risk evaluation based on purely genetic or demographic information, as done here, has to be completed by socio-economic factors or other considerations peculiar to each country. Anyhow, the situation points out to the need for a regional co-ordination in defining conservation strategies (Ollivier, 1998). Such a regional co-ordination is indeed an important element of the FAO Global Strategy mentioned earlier (see 2.).

Comparisons of successive inventories in the course of time are also of interest for evaluating trends in number of breeds currently exploited and possible changes in the proportion of breeds in each category of endangerment. In the European pig over the last 20 years, such comparisons show that breed extinction has been largely avoided, at least among those breeds listed in the initial inventories. As an example it can be seen, by going back to the list of critically endangered breeds in Simon and Buchenauer (1993 p. 66) that the 9 native breeds listed in that category are still existing presently, and it is also worth noting that 4 of them are no more critically endangered.

5. Conclusion

This overview has shown the need for a better understanding of the nature of the world pig genetic resources. FAO has recently been entrusted with the co-ordination of an evaluation of the state of the world animal genetic resources, a process which should extend over the period 2000-2005 (Scherf, 2000). An impressive amount of information has indeed been collected all over the world during the last 20 years. As we have seen, some clear priorities can be defined for regions such as Asia, Latin America or Tropical Africa. The European situation is also well documented. A list of Uniform Resource Locators (URL) containing information on European pig breeds is given in the Appendix. It should be stressed that the information presented on those URLs very much reflects the data provided by each country. In spite of the efforts made to co-ordinate the inventories across different countries, the data should not be considered as necessarily representing comprehensive coverage of all situations, as we have seen above for the European pig genetic resources. Much remains to be done to improve the quality of the information needed for the most efficient use of pig genetic resources throughout the world. Improving information quality is indeed one of the main purposes of the following chapters of this book, devoted to 4 major pig producing countries of the European Union.

Acknowledgement

The authors are grateful to the Food and Agriculture Organisation of the United Nations for its permission to reproduce part of the pages 177-187 and tables 1 and 2 from the FAO Animal Production and Health paper no 104 (Hodges J. (ed.), 1992).

Appendix: List of some Uniform Resource Locators (URL) containing information on breeds of farm animals in Europe

Institution	URL
FAO DAD-IS[1]	http://www.fao.org/dad-is
EAAP-AGDB[2]	http://www.tiho-hannover.de/einricht/zucht/eaap/index.htm
NGB[3]	http://www.nordgen.org/english/engindex.html
BRG[4]	http://www.brg.prd.fr/
SERGA[5]	http://www.uco.es/organiza/departamentos/genetica/serga/

[1]Food and Agriculture Organisation, Domestic Animal Diversity Information System, Rome, Italy.
[2]European Association for Animal Production Animal Genetic Data Bank, School of Veterinary Medicine, Hanover, Germany.
[3]Nordic Gene Bank, Aas, Norway.
[4]Bureau des Ressources Génétiques, Paris, France.
[5]Spanish Society for Animal Genetic Resources, Cordoba, Spain.

Chapter 1.2. Pig genetic resources of France

F. Labroue[1], M. Luquet[1], H. Marsac[1], I. Canope[2], D. Rinaldo[3] and L. Ollivier[4]

[1]*ITP, Pôle Amélioration de l'Animal, BP 3, 35651 Le Rheu Cedex, France,*
[2]*INRA., Station d'Amélioration Génétique des Animaux, BP 27, 31326 Castanet Tolosan, France*
[3]*INRA, Unité de recherches zootechniques, 97170 Petit-Bourg, Guadeloupe*
[4]*INRA., Station de Génétique Quantitative et Appliquée, 78352 Jouy-en-Josas Cedex, France*

1. Organisation of pig genetic resources in France

A conservation programme of local breeds of pig has been set up in France in 1981 at the request of the French Ministry of Agriculture (Labroue and Luquet, 1999). It associates 2 main actors: ITP (Pig Technical Institute) and INRA. The aims are as follows:
- to update the inventory of the different local breeds and maintain within-breed genetic variability through a strict management of mating,
- to search for possibilities of drawing economic benefits from those breeds by studying the genetic specificities of each breed, and especially to carry out experiments in INRA stations in order to measure production traits.

The LIGERAL Association, in charge of collectively managing the herd books of local breeds, was created in 1996, and received the official agreement of the French Ministry of Agriculture. The members of LIGERAL are the breeders' associations, and ITP and INRA as associated organisations. The main missions of LIGERAL are:
- to define the trends of each breed's preservation programme,
- to bring the preservation programme of each breed into operation,
- to control the reliability of the information provided by the breeders,
- to manage the herd book of each breed,
- to deliver the certificates of origin of purebred sows and boars,
- to manage the admission of boars in AI centres,
- and more generally to carry out any kind of action leading to a better knowledge of each local breed.

All actions of genetic management have been delegated by LIGERAL to ITP. A national data base has been created in order to collect all the information provided by the breeders (see paragraph 2). One of the most important genetic missions consists in maintaining a wide range of boars in activity either by creating special farms to raise entire males before sending them to breeders or by using stocks of frozen semen under strictly controlled conditions. The management of within-breed variability is also delegated to ITP. The evolution of inbreeding is regularly estimated and kinship coefficients between sows and boars are supplied to local technicians and breeders in order to avoid mating between close relatives.

2. The local breeds database

Since 1996, a computerised database has been collecting the information on 5 French local pig breeds: *Basque* (BA), *Blanc de l'Ouest* (BO), *Bayeux* (BY), *Gascon* (GA) and *Limousin* (LI). The chronological record of data stored at ITP since 1981, the beginning of the national preservation programme, has been integrated into the database which today records about 5400 breeding animals and 5600 litters (Marsac *et al.*, 1999).

2.1. Information stored in the database

Data concerning local breeds are stored in 3 tables:

- Table «Breeders» containing all data related to each breeder (name, first name, address, breed of animals, breeding timetable...).
- Table «Animals» containing all data related to each animal (national identification, birth date, sire identification, dam identification, breeder, date of entry, date of culling).
- Since 1997, following the creation of the collective herd books of local breeds (LIGERAL), the identification of all purebred piglets has become a legal obligation. The identification numbers of piglets are also stored in the table «Animals».
- Table «Litters» containing all data related to each litter (dam identification, date of farrowing, sire identification, parity, numbers of total born, born alive, and weaned piglets...).

2.2. Links with other databases

Each year, the information stored to the database is used to update the French national database of animal genetic resources of BRG (http://www.brg.prd.fr/). From this national database, two international databases are also updated: the European database of EAAP and the world database of FAO, available for consultation at the following websites:
http://www.tiho-hannover.de/einricht/zucht/eaap/index.htm
http://www.fao.org/dad-is/

3. Evolution of population sizes over the past 5 years

The evolution of population sizes has been fully described by Marsac *et al.* (1999). The evolution of the number of sows per breed over the past 5 years is given in table 1. Whatever the breed, the number of sows increased. The most important increase (60%) was observed in *Blanc de l'Ouest*, but the 4 other breeds also showed a considerable increase of the number of sows (46%, 45%, 37% et 36% for *Gascon*, *Basque*, *Bayeux* and *Limousin*, respectively).

Table 1. Numbers of sows, boars and farms per breed and per year.

Breed	Traits	1995	1996	1997	1998	1999
Basque	Nb. of sows	131	115	146	193	240
	Nb. of boars	40	25	25	32	54
	Nb. of farms	19	22	23	29	33
Blanc de l'Ouest	Nb. of sows	49	60	82	128	123
	Nb. of boars	19	20	25	41	34
	Nb. of farms	21	23	30	39	38
Bayeux	Nb. of sows	43	58	67	67	68
	Nb. of boars	12	17	21	17	22
	Nb. of farms	16	20	24	24	31
Gascon	Nb. of sows	173	190	232	271	320
	Nb. of boars	38	44	55	65	70
	Nb. of farms	61	64	78	78	77
Limousin	Nb. of sows	94	120	145	148	148
	Nb. of boars	25	32	40	45	48
	Nb. of farms	27	34	35	37	41

The evolution of the number of boars per breed over the past 5 years is given in table 1. This number increases whatever the breed, and the classification between breeds is the same as for the number of sows. However, the mating ratio, *i.e.* the number of sows per boar, was higher (about 4.5) in *Gascon* and *Basque* (the two largest breeds in size) than in the three other breeds (only 3 sows per boar on average). The ideal number, in order to minimise inbreeding, would be one sow per boar on average.

The evolution of the number of farms per breed over the past 5 years is given in table 1. The increase observed was far less important here than for the numbers of breeding animals, which means that the increase of the total population size was rather due to an increase of the size of the existing farms than to the setting up of new farms. In addition, the classification between breeds was not the same as for the numbers of breeding animals, because the average farm size differed from one breed to another.

4. The French continental local breeds

The 5 French local breeds listed in section 2 above are included in the national conservation programme (I.T.P., 1999). These five breeds were all included in the RESGEN12 project and, with the exception of BY, they were also included in the PiGMaP pilot diversity study.

Table 2. Geographic location of the French continental local breeds (1999 situation).

Breed	Department	Nb. of sows	Nb. of boars	Nb. of farms	Nb. of sows per farm
Basque	Pyrénées Atlantique	194	41	19	10.2
	Hautes Pyrénées	35	8	6	5.8
	Others	11	5	8	1.4
	Total	**240**	**54**	**33**	**7.3**
Blanc de l'Ouest	Calvados	30	10	5	6.0
	Côtes d'Armor	33	9	7	4.7
	Finistère	10	1	4	2.5
	Ille et Vilaine	13	3	3	4.3
	Loire Atlantique	10	2	5	2.0
	Others	27	9	14	1.9
	Total	**123**	**34**	**38**	**3.2**
Bayeux	Calvados	24	7	11	2.2
	Maine-et-Loir	14	2	1	14.0
	Others	30	13	19	1.6
	Total	**68**	**22**	**31**	**2.2**
Gascon	Ariège	32	7	9	3.6
	Gers	59	9	10	5.9
	Hautes-Pyrénées	141	34	29	4.9
	Others	88	20	29	3.0
	Total	**320**	**70**	**77**	**4.2**
Limousin	Corrèze	17	4	6	2.8
	Dordogne	20	13	6	3.3
	Haute-Vienne	92	25	20	4.6
	Others	19	6	9	2.1
	Total	**148**	**48**	**41**	**3.6**

4.1. Basque (BA)

Origin and distribution
The *Basque* breed used to live in the west of the *Pyrénées* and in the north of Spain. Several varieties could be identified:
- the *Béarnaise* variety, rather black than white, with a thin body and long limbs.
- the *Basque* variety, with shorter limbs, a compact body and no black spot in the middle of the back.
- the *Bigourdane* variety, strong and sturdy, with black head, black bottom, and a black spot on the back. This third variety, which resulted from various crossings with a Celtic breed, has nearly disappeared now.

The *Basque* herd book was founded in 1921. Due to its resistance to bad climatic conditions, its low food requirements and its adaptation to extensive breeding, the breed is very well adapted to mountain breeding. The decreasing number of oaks, due to uncontrolled deforestation by shepherds looking for new pastures, led to the almost total disappearance of the breed.
   Today, BA pigs can mainly be found in *Pyrénées Atlantiques* (near Bayonne) and *Hautes Pyrénées* (near Tarbes). With 240 sows and 54 boars, raised in 33 farms, the BA breed is the second French local breed as regards its global size. The breeding area is mainly located in the *Aquitaine* region (83% of sows). The geographic location of the breed is given in table 2.

Breed standard (see plate 2)
The head is long and right in profile with a mobile snout. The limbs are strong and long. The *Basque* pig has a black pied coat (black head and rear end) with large and well delimited spots. In adults, the height at the withers is 0.75 m and body length 1.4 m.

Breed exploitation
The *Basque* pig has built the reputation of *Bayonne* ham in the past centuries. This free range pig is able to feed in woods as well as in fields. When slaughtered between 12 and 15 months of age, it then weighs 120 to 160 kg. Once this live weight has been reached, the fat is not too thick and the full-flavoured flesh is well adapted to delicatessen (charcuterie) production and dry ham processing. Since 1994, the *Basque* production has been organized with a network of breeders (producing weaned piglets and/or slaughter pigs) all supplying the same traditional salting firm with carcasses of purebred animals. The prices have been fixed in agreement with breeders in a range of 13 F/kg to 24 F/kg depending on both carcass weight and back fat thickness. Breeders also have to respect several breeding conditions (extensive fattening, minimum age at slaughter,...). The present production is above 2000 pigs slaughtered per year, aiming at 3000 pigs per year for 2000.

4.2. Blanc de l'Ouest (BO)

Origin and distribution
The origin goes back to the Celtic type of pig which used to live in the west of France at the end of the Middle Age. It was tall, with a flat snout and drooping ears. From *Flandres* to Brittany, it was known under different names: *Flamand, Boulonnais, Normand* or *Craonnais*. Until 1958, the last two populations could still be identified:
- the *Normand* breed with a breeders' association founded in December 1937 and located in Saint Hilaire-du-Harcouët (Manche),
- the *Craonnais* breed with a herd book founded in 1926 and located in Craon (*Mayenne*).

The merging of these two breeds under the name of *Blanc de l'Ouest*, operated on May 1958 (Quittet and Zert, 1971), did not allow anymore, at least in theory, to distinguish *Normand* from *Craonnais* pig. However, the two genetic types still exist. Ten years later, the introduction of *Veredeltes Landschwein* from Germany, in order to improve sow prolificacy, led to the disappearance of a large part of the original breed. However, a few breeders refused to introduce *Veredeltes Landschwein* in their herds. They saved the breed from a complete extinction.

Today, BO pigs can mainly be found in Brittany (*Côtes d'Armor*, *Ille et Vilaine* and *Finistère*) and in a few farms located in Normandy (*Calvados*) and *Pays de la Loire* (*Loire-Atlantique*). With 123 sows and 34 boars, raised in 38 farms, the BO breed is the fourth French local breed as regards its global size. The breeding area is mainly located in Brittany and Normandy (84% of sows). The geographic location of the breed is given in table 2.

Breed standard (see plate 4)
The *Blanc de l'Ouest* pig has a white coat with a whorl on the back, a head of average length and a concave profile. The large ears droop and cover the eyes. In adults, height at the withers is 1.05-1.10 m, body length 1.70-1.90 m, weight 350 kg in sows and 400 kg in boars.

Breed exploitation
The *Blanc de l'Ouest* pig is well adapted to outdoor breeding. The prolificacy is medium but piglets are heavy and precocious. The good quality meat is known for its aptitude to delicatessen production. The breed offers 3 main types of incomes: suckling pigs sold to restaurants, home made delicatessen directly sold on farms, and purebred sows and boars sold for crossbreeding with selected lines. The latter type tends to increase, especially with new quality labels becoming popular, such as the «red label» or organic production. An experiment is being carried out in order to test slaughter pigs with 25% of BO genes. The first step, at present in progress, consists in producing F1 boars (50% BO) that will be mated with sows of selected maternal lines.

4.3. Bayeux (BY)

Origin and distribution
The *Bayeux* pig originates from crosses performed in the middle of the 19th century between the *Normand* and the English *Berkshire* pigs. The small region around Bayeux called *Bessin* (*Calvados*) is the original breeding area and, before the second world war, the *Bayeux* pig could be found in almost all farms of Normandy. The *Bayeux* pig was one of the first French breeds admitted in «official herd books register».

This large sized pig, called «concave type with drooping ears» has a long and thick body and a strong head. The alternate variant «*Longué* pig» (*Maine-et-Loire*), resulting from crosses between *Craonnais* and *Berkshire*, is similar to *Bayeux* pig for coat and conformation, but the head is shorter and more concave, with a stronger and shorter snout.

The *Bayeux* herd book was founded in 1928, and located in *Bayeux* (*Calvados*). In 1944, the Allies' landing decimated the herds and the breeders had to restore their strains. In the 1960s the *Bayeux* herd book was reorganised with the legal obligation to declare farrowings and to identify piglets before weaning.

Today, BY pigs can mainly be found in a few farms located in *Calvados* and *Maine-et-Loire*. With 68 sows and 22 boars, raised in 31 farms, the BY breed is the smallest French local breed in global size. The breeding area is mainly located in the *Normandie* and *Pays de la Loire* regions (74% of sows). The geographic location of the breed is given in table 2.

Breed standard (see plate 3)
The *Bayeux* pig has a white coat with large round patches, a head of average length and a concave profile. The thin ears are medium in size, horizontal or sometimes slightly drooping. The trunk is long and thick with right pads. In adults, the height at the withers is 0.90 m, and weight 350 kg.

Breed exploitation
This outdoor pig is very well adapted to a feeding based on dairy by-products. The sows have a medium prolificacy but good maternal abilities. The Bayeux production is being organised with the financial support of both the Conservatory of Normandie and the city of Bayeux. The aim is to synchronise farrowings among the present breeders in order to constitute batches of 20-25 piglets. These piglets are bought by new breeders for fattening under strict conditions (outdoor breeding, feeding using dairy by products,...). The first year is dedicated to the elaboration of a feeding programme and the study of production traits. The first batch of 25 pigs started control in June 2000 and will be slaughtered in October 2000.

4.4. Gascon (GA)

Origin and distribution
The *Gascon* pig, of Iberian type, is solid black and originates from *Piémont Pyrénéen*. The original breeding area is located in the small region of *Nébouzan* wedged between *Armagnac*, *Comminges* and *Lomagne*. According to Professor Girard (1921, Veterinary review), the *Gascon* pig breed could be the oldest type of pig known in France.
    Two varieties are known:
- the *Tournayaise* (area of *Tournay*) with rather short ears and sharp-pointed nose,
- the *Bleue de Boulogne* (*Boulogne-sur-Gesse*) with drooping ears, a slightly turned-up nose and shining hair (bluish hair). For a long time, the main centre for *Gascon* pigs was the area of *Boulogne-sur-Gesse*.

The *Gascon* breed has been crossed with improved breeds, which led to the *Cazères* pigs (*Gascon* x *Large White*) and the *Miélan* pigs (*Gascon* x *Craonnais*), better adapted to modern breeding conditions (Quittet and Zert, 1971). However, these «crossbred breeds» have now totally disappeared. A few purebred sows found in 1981 allowed to save the breed. Until 1992, ITP contributed to this rescue, by creating a multiplication farm of 5 boars and 10 sows in order to provide boars to the breeders.
    Today, GA pigs can mainly be found in a few farms located in *Hautes-Pyrénées* and *Gers*. With 320 sows and 70 boars, raised in 77 farms, the GA breed is the largest French local breed in global size. The breeding area is mainly located in the *Midi-Pyrénées* region (80% of sows). The geographic location of the breed is given in table 2.

Breed standard (see plate 5)
The *Gascon* pig has a solid black coat with long and hard hair. The head is long and thin with a sharp-pointed face. The thin ears are horizontal and slightly sloping above the eyes. The rather compact body is somewhat cylindrical. In adults, the height at the withers is 0.75 m, body length 1.20 m, weight 350 kg in sows and 400 kg in boars.

Breed exploitation
The *Gascon* pig is rustic and sturdy. It can withstand heat and easily feed on pastures. Its growth is rather slow: it weighs only 100 kg at one year of age. The fat is firm and the meat of a good quality is well adapted to dry ham processing. Since 1997, the *Gascon* production has

been organised with a network of breeders, producers-transformers, pork butchers and one salting firm. The prices have been fixed in agreement with breeders in a range of 12 F/kg to 20 F/kg depending on both carcass weight and back fat thickness. The present production is above 1000 pigs slaughtered per year, aiming at 3000 pigs per year for 2000.

4.5. Limousin (LI)

Origin and distribution
The *Limousin* pig, of Iberian type, also called *Saint-Yrieix*, or «Cul Noir» (referring to its coat colour pattern), has been living for several centuries in the west of *Massif Central*, where it has been known since the 16th century. Around 1850, two varieties existed, mainly differing in size:
- the variety called «little breed», with chubby shapes, very high ribs and right ears pointing high forwards.
- the other variety is larger, with a thinner body, stronger and more horizontal ears, and generally more hair.

This distinction disappeared in the 1900's, except for a part of the second variety, which crossed with *Craonnais*, led to the *Périgourdin* breed, with a herd book founded in 1931. The *Limousin* herd book was founded in September 1935 and located in St Yrieix-la-Perche.

The herd books were discontinued during the war 1940-45 and never started their activity again. This phenomenon, combined with the introduction of «modern» breeds, explains the large decrease of animal numbers in both breeds (13000 sows in 1953 *vs.* a few hundred in 1970).

Today, pigs of both *Limousin* and *Périgourdin* types are in the same herd book. The breeders are mainly settled in the area of *Saint Yrieix* (*Hte-Vienne*), *Lanouailles* (*Dordogne*) and *Ségur-le-Château* (*Corrèze*). The breeding area is mainly located in the *Limousin* region (82% of sows). The geographic location of the breed is given in table 2.

Breed standard (see plate 6)
The *Limousin* pig has a black pied coat (black head and rear end) with large and well delimited spots. It is a pig of medium size, with a compact and cylindrical body, a head right in profile and thin ears pointing forwards. In adults, height at the withers is 0.8 m.

Breed exploitation
The *Limousin* pig is a rustic animal with a rather slow growth. It is known for the quality of both its meat and fat. The lard type pig is slaughtered after the chestnut season in November or December. It is then 18 months old and can weigh up to 170 to 230 kg. The breed offers 2 main types of income: either home made delicatessen directly sold on farms, or purebred carcasses sold to pork butchers, particularly just before Christmas. A third possible source of income could be purebred sows and boars used in crossbreeding with selected lines. This income could become more important with new quality labels such as the «red label». An experiment is being carried out in order to test slaughter pigs with 25% of LI genes. The first step, at present in progress, consists in producing F1 boars (50% LI) that will be mated with sows of selected maternal lines.

5. The French over-sea department of Guadeloupe: the particular case of the Créole pig (CR)

Origin and distribution
The *Créole* pig (CR) is described as resulting from a cross between Iberian stocks introduced into West-Indies as early as the 16th century and French pigs which were brought in at the same time with this country colonisation (Dutertre, 1667-1671; Labat, 1722). The original local population has been widely crossbred throughout centuries, following the introduction of British (*Large Black*, *Yorkshire*), American (*Duroc*, *Hampshire*) and French (*Normand*, *Craonnais*) breeds. As a result, CR is today a highly polymorphic pig population (Lauvergne and Canope, 1979) with a high variation in size, production level (Canope and Raynaud, 1980 and 1981) and colour patterns, though the caryotypes of the European and CR pigs were found to be similar (2n=38, as shown by Popescu *et al.,* 1989). The total number of CR sows is 1200, distributed over Basse-Terre (50%), Grande-Terre (33%) and the nearby island of Marie-Galante (17%).

Breed standard (see plate 7)
Under traditional husbandry conditions, *Créole* pig is lanky and long-limbed with silky bristle: the lankier the pig, the silkier the bristle. CR also shows a long snout. Colour pattern variants are, however, the only and best way of discriminating CR pig varieties. Four of them are the most commonly observed: silky black, «domino» *i.e.* black and red, grey (roan) and «chabin» (dirty white coat).

Organization of conservation
A new breeders' association (SOS-PIG: Sauvegarde Organisée et Sélection du Porc Indigène de Guadeloupe) is playing a significant role in the promotion of the Guadeloupe endangered indigenous pig (CR), with the co-operation of both INRA and local pig breeders. Experiments carried on from 1976 to 1980 showed several assets of the female CR, namely early puberty and successful mating, at about 6 and 7 months respectively, leading to an annual CR sow productivity of 13.8 piglets / year *vs.* 14.6 for Large White kept in the same tropical conditions. Later analyses gave significant productivity improvement (2.7 piglets) and showed specific optimum slaughter weights, namely 65 kg for CR *vs.* 85 kg for Large White. A detailed review on reproduction, growth and meat quality traits in relation to dietary conditions has been recently published by Rinaldo *et al.* (2000).

Breed exploitation
The CR pig is known for its hardiness and adaptation to extremely harsh rural environment. This advantage has been exploited for the benefit of Haitian farmers, when their country had to be restocked after the outbreak of African swine fever in 1983. The use of a combination of the CR pig of Guadeloupe, the GA pig described in 4.4. and highly prolific Chinese breeds (Taihu) has quickly provided genotypes well adapted to Haitian conditions. They were in particular able to maintain satisfactory reproductive capacities under the most unfavourable farm husbandry conditions (Delatte *et al.,* 1991).

6. Within-breed genetic variability

A retrospective study of genetic variability in each local breed was performed at the end of year 1998 on the base of genealogical data. Two methods were used: inbreeding and probabilities of gene origin (founders, effective founders and effective ancestors). The reference population included all females born between 1996 and 1998 with both parents known.

6.1. Pedigree completeness

At least 3 criteria highlight the completeness of the pedigrees for the 5 local breeds (see fig.1):
- more than 90% of ancestry were still known at generation 4,
- the threshold of 50% was crossed only at generation 8 or later,
- for a few animals, the pedigrees went back 20 generations, which is exceptional and corresponds to founders born in the 1950s.

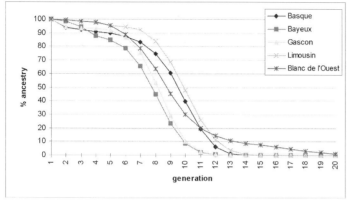

Figure 1. Representation of pedigree completeness.

6.2. Probabilities of gene origin

Three numbers of founders are given in table 3:
1. The total number of founders *i.e.* the missing information at the beginning of the pedigrees for all animals of the reference population. These are also called «computer» founders because they correspond to the beginning of computerised data sets. The number of founders was in a range of 148 for *Blanc de l'Ouest* to 18 for *Bayeux*. This illustrates the within breed genetic variability at the beginning of data recording.
2. The number of effective founders *i.e.* a theoretical number of founders assuming that all of them equally contribute to the reference population. In other words, the difference between founders and effective founders illustrates the unbalanced contributions of the different founders. The most unbalanced contributions were observed for *Blanc de l'Ouest* (only 24.4 effective founders for 148 founders) and to a lesser extent for *Basque* (10.7 effective founders for 44 founders). For the three other breeds, the number of effective founders was about half the number of founders.
3. The number of effective ancestors, which takes into account the bottlenecks in pedigrees. The difference between effective founders and effective ancestors illustrates the frequency of bottlenecks in pedigrees. *Limousin* had the highest frequency, followed by *Gascon* and *Blanc de l'Ouest*. As regards *Basque* and *Bayeux* however, the difference between effective founders and ancestors was very small, which means there were few bottlenecks in pedigrees. According to the number of effective ancestors, the largest breed was *Blanc de l'Ouest*, followed by *Gascon, Basque, Limousin* and *Bayeux*. This ranking of *Blanc de l'Ouest* appeared to be different from the one based on actual population size, though the four other breeds ranked in the same order using the 2 criteria (see table 1).

Table 3. Numbers of founders, effective founders and effective ancestors.

Breed	Reference population			Founders	Effective founders	Effective ancestors
	sex	birth period	nb. animals			
Basque	F	96 - 98	359	44	10.70	9.63
Bayeux	F	96 - 98	97	18	9.40	7.44
Blanc de l'Ouest	F	96 - 98	280	148	24.40	18.50
Gascon	F	96 - 98	902	44	20.30	14.18
Limousin	F	96 - 98	328	33	15.20	8.88

A second approach of probabilities of gene origin is the evaluation of the main ancestors respective contributions. They are given in table 4. According to these results, *Bayeux* and *Limousin* had the lowest genetic variability with only 3 ancestors contributing for 50% of genes of the reference population. Then came *Gascon*, *Basque* and *Blanc de l'Ouest*. The ranking of breeds was exactly the same as with the number of effective ancestors. The main ancestors respective contributions were just another way of illustrating the same phenomenon.

Table 4. Main ancestors' respective contributions.

Breed	Contribution of the main ancestor	Contribution of the 5 main ancestors	Contribution of the 10 main ancestors	Number of ancestors explaining 50% of genes
Basque	21%	65%	84%	4
Bayeux	24%	75%	96%	3
Blanc de l'Ouest	12%	43%	64%	7
Gascon	13%	51%	75%	5
Limousin	21%	69%	85%	3

6.3. Inbreeding

The average inbreeding level ranged from 8% in *Blanc de l'Ouest* to 18% in Bayeux (table 5). Again, the ranking of breeds according to the average inbreeding level is the same as with effective ancestors: the highest number of effective founders was found in the breed with the lowest average inbreeding level.

Table 5. Inbreeding results.

Breed	Reference population size	Average inbreeding level
Basque	359	11.99 %
Bayeux	97	17.96 %
Blanc de l'Ouest	280	7.62 %
Gascon	902	8.96 %
Limousin	328	14.33 %

Fig. 2 clearly illustrates the differences between breeds as regards the average inbreeding level. In addition, the evolution of the average inbreeding level from 1980 to 1998 illustrates the three main trends observed:

1. For *Basque* and *Gascon*, the rate of increase was lower after 1990 than before, despite the relatively low number of founders at the beginning (only 44). This demonstrates an efficient genetic management, in particular in the use of planned matings.
2. For *Blanc de l'Ouest*, the rate of increase was rather low, but probably because this breed had the highest genetic variability at the beginning, with 128 founders.
3. For *Bayeux* and *Limousin*, the population size increased and so did the average inbreeding level. The genetic variability at the beginning was however already lower for these two breeds, according to the number of founders (18 and 33 for *Bayeux* and *Limousin*, respectively).

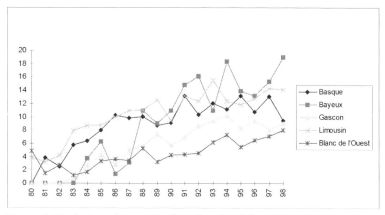

Figure 2. Evolution of average inbreeding level from 1980 to 1998.

Chapter 1.3. Pig genetic resources of Germany[1]

P. Glodek

Institute of Animal Breeding and Genetics, University of Göttingen, Albrecht-Thaer-Weg 3, 37075 Göttingen, Germany

1. Changes of pig genetic resources in the period of pedigree recording

Pedigree pig breeding organisations were founded in Germany more than 100 years ago, and they started with a diverse mixture of unimproved local strains and original import pigs from many British breeds (*Large* and *Middle White, Berkshire, Poland China, Cornwall* and *Tamworth*). But pure British breeds declined and were increasingly utilised in crossing and upgrading of the local breeds. So in the early 20th century four more or less consolidated German breed groups were developed and presented at national DLG-shows besides the two remaining British breeds *Cornwall* and *Berkshire* (Comberg, 1978): *Deutsches Edelschwein* (DE), *Veredeltes Landschwein* or *Landrace* (DvL), *Schwäbisch-Hällisches Schwein* (SH), *Angler Sattelschwein* (AS) and *Weideschwein* (DW). These breeds survived both world wars without much genetic improvement, despite of the station tests introduced from 1927 on, and were still available as genetic resources in 1950. But from then on, as a result of consumer demand turning from fat to lean meat, drastic changes in the German breed composition occurred as table 1 shows.

Table 1. Registered pedigree animals and breeds in Germany 1953 vs. 1998.

Breed names	1953[1]		1998	
	n	%	n	%
Landrace (DvL)	16 778	67.0	36 758	61.6
Schwäbisch-Hällisches Schwein (SH)	2 763	11.0	215	0.4
Angler/Deutsches Sattelschwein (AS/DS)	2 707	10.8	304	0.5
Deutsches Edelschwein (DE/LW)	1 491	6.0	8 145	13.6
Bunte Bentheimer (BB)	291	1.2	55	0.1
Weideschwein (DW)	494	2.0	(until 1971)	
Cornwall (DC)	374	1.5	(until 1961)	
Rotbunte (Rbt)	138	0.6	(until 1970)	
Piétrain (PI)	(since 1961)		11 720	19.6
Leicoma (Lc)[2]	(since 1989)		1.576	2.6
Duroc (DU)	(since 1982)		406	0.7
Belgian Landrace (LB)	(since 1971)		332	0.6
Hampshire (HA)	(since 1983)		169	0.3
No. (Breeds) Pedigree Animals	(8)	25 036	(10)	59 680

[1]West Germany only; [2]DDR-Synthetic.

---

[1] Two breeds from neighbouring countries of Germany were also included in the RESGEN project, namely the Czech *Presticke* (see plate 12) and the Polish *Pulawska* (see plate 13) breeds, on which references are given at the end of this book.

Although the number of pedigree breeds kept was greater in 1998 than in 1953, two local breeds (DW, Rbt) and the original British fat breeds (*Cornwall* and *Berkshire*) were lost forever, and also the BB and SH breeds lost their pedigree status but were revived later. Instead, four new Western meat type breeds (PI, DU, LB, HA) which were used as terminal sires in various hybrid programmes, and one synthetic dam breed developed in East Germany, (Lc) were newly introduced.

While the *Weideschwein* (DW), as the last local breed adapted to extensive forest and pasture production, became extinct with the last remaining herd in South Hannover in 1971 the two Saddlebacks (AS, SH) and the *Bunte Bentheimer* (BB) are still the most endangered genetic resource populations in Germany, whose conservation is subsidised by regional public sources since the mid 1980s. All these populations were hardy local breeds with the highest litter performance under extensive production conditions in 1950, but all three were inferior to the *Landrace* standard in carcass composition and lean content, as shown in table 2.

Table 2. Comparison of endangered breeds with the DvL (Landrace) standard in the 1950's.

	Trait	AS/DS	SH	BB	DvL-Standard
Litter recording, 1955/56	No sows recorded	1544	2256	220	14677
	No litters per sow and year	1.90	1.90	2.00	1.90
	No pigs born per litter	11.10	11.80	12.00	10.80
	No pigs weaned per litter	9.50	10.00	10.20	9.00
	No pigs born per sow and year	21.70	22.60	23.70	20.90
	No pigs weaned per sow and year	18.40	19.10	20.30	17.50
Fattening and carcass traits at station test (40 -100 kg), 1958	No. groups (2 males/2 females)	40	38	21*	1319
	Daily gain (g)	720	716	722	718
	Feed conversion (kg)	3.65	3.48	3.66	3.60
	Carcass length (cm)	96.50	92.90	93.40	94.80
	Backfat thickness (mm)	47	47	47	46
	Loin eye area (cm^2)	26.30	25.90	-	29.70
	Lean-fat area ratio	2.07	1.87	-	1.64

*BB 1954-60.

This disadvantage increased in the following years when other breeds were improved rapidly by upgrading with *Dutch Landrace* (Glodek, 1963) and with the introduction of Belgian meaty breeds to Germany.

2. Management of pig genetic resources in Germany

Farm animal breeding as well as the conservation of animal genetic resources, although ruled by a federal legislature (the animal breeding law or Tierzuchtgesetz TZG) is executed under the responsibility of twelve State Ministries of Agriculture which usually have delegated the pedigree registration and breed management to recognised breed societies of the same species in the region. Through these also financial subsidies are given to breeders who participate in recognised conservation programmes, but the States apply different subsidy schemes even if they support the same breed. So the BB, located in the Weser-Ems Region of Niedersachsen is subsidised by the Hannover Government, the SH, concentrated in Württemberg, by its Ministry in Stuttgart. The AS population originates in Angeln/Schleswig-Holstein and is supported by this State. Under the name DS the former East German Saddleback population, originating from AS and SH herds located there, is distributed over all five New States and subsidised by some of these (Ehlich, 1997).

In addition, the "Gesellschaft für die Erhaltung bedrohter Haustierrassen (GEH)", a NGO dedicated to endangered farm animal breeds, supports many conservation projects by providing honorary breed tutors and grants from ist sponsor money (GEH/Hörning, 1997).

The scientific supervision of such programmes in recent years was provided by a Committee of the Deutsche Gesellschaft für Züchtungskunde which has published a series of papers on its activities in vols. 66-70 of "Züchtungskunde".

The collection and storage of all data on German farm animal breeds is done in the EAAP-data bank at the Tierärztliche Hochschule in Hanover (Simon and Buchenauer, 1993) which also transfers the data regularly into the FAO Domestic Animal Diversity-Information System (DAD-IS). The German Focal Point of the FAO-DAD-programme is the IGR-ZADI agency at the Federal Ministry of Agriculture in Bonn (see IGR/ZADI and Oetman, 2000).

3. The present pig resource populations in Germany

3.1. Saddleback Populations

At present in Germany three more or less related Saddleback populations are registered under different names in different regional pedigree breed societies:
  Angler Sattelschwein (AS: see plate 8);
  Deutsches Sattelschwein (DS: see plate 9);
  Schwäbisch-Hällisches Schwein (SH: see plate 10).

SH and AS are old German breeds which were developed from unimproved local breeds with some British *Wessex* imports in the Angeln region in Schleswig-Holstein (Haring, 1961) and in the Schwäbisch Hall region in Württemberg (Bühler, 1987; Kober, 1992). Regular boar exchanges between both populations started in the 1920's and both reached their largest expansion all over Germany in world war two because of their high fat production ability from non food sources. Although AS was continuously represented in the German pedigree breed statistics (see table 1), Glodek *et al.* (1990) showed that it changed its genetic composition very markedly over the years 1950 to 1990.

DS originated from combining the AS and SH pedigree herds located in the Soviet sector in 1948. In 1968 the DS pedigree breeding was discontinued in the DDR and the remaining DS pigs were maintained pure as the "DS-gene reserve" in only one large farm (Hirschfeld) in Sachsen and utilized in breeding the *Leicoma* Synthetic (Pfeiffer, 1980). This herd was disbanded in 1990 but many breeding animals were sold to small (often ecological) farms all over Germany. Breeding herds were registered in four of the five East German State pig herdbooks as DS. In West Germany the imported DS-breeding animals were directly registered in the AS and SH herdbooks.

In 1991 all Saddleback breeders founded the "Arbeitsgemeinschaft Deutscher Sattelschweinzüchter (AGDS)" which meets yearly to discuss breeding and maintenance activities. In 1993 this group defined an uniform breeding goal for all German Saddlebacks and accepted the free exchange of stock among them, but the separate breed names and herdbooks were still maintained. Mathes (1996) analysed the breeding policies and genetic relationships of the three strains and concluded that the genetic distance between them would further decrease very rapidly by the new breeding policy. But shortly after the German reunification Glodek *et al.* (1993) estimated the genetic distances between 5 East and 6 West German pig breeds, among them the 3 Saddleback strains, using 71 allele frequencies of blood polymorphisms (13 blood groups, 5 serum and 4 enzyme systems), and came up with the figures in table 3.

Table 3. Degree of heterozygosity and genetic distance between German Saddleback strains (Glodek et al. 1993).

Strain	n	Degree of heterozygosity	Genetic distance* DS	SH
AS	171	36.0 (102)**	2.55 (86)	2.43 (82)
DS	349	33.8 (96)	-	2.98 (100)
SH	134	36.7 (104)	-	-

*distance of Gregorius (1974); **in brackets: in % of means over 11 breeds.

These figures show the lowest heterozygosity in DS, which is explained by their 20 year closed breeding in one gene reserve herd. AS and SH, although kept in very small populations for many years, are much more variable because of frequent immigrations from several other breeds, as has been shown by Glodek *et al.* (1990) for AS. Genetic distances indicate that AS already in 1990 was closely related to DS and SH, whereas for the latter two only an average relationship was found. This is explained by the described breed histories up to 1990 but the differences have disappeared by the combined actions since then.

In summary, the three herdbook populations AS, DS and SH, still registered under these three names in six regional breed societies, are closely related strains of one German Saddleback breed. It would, therefore, not only be genetically justified but also helpful to most of their future breeding and conservation activities if they were combined in one national herdbook under one name (Glodek, 2000).

3.2. Bunte Bentheimer

This breed (see plate 11) was always more or less restricted to the Bentheim region and therefore did not reach nearly the importance of Saddlebacks in German pig production. It originated in the region from spotted local pigs (*Wettringer Tigerschweine*) and reached its peak population size in the 1920s before the TZG made boar licensing obligatory. With the introduction of the TZG the BB was not officially recognised as pedigree breed and therefore the use of BB boars became illegal (Schröder, 1997). Only in 1950 this ban on BB boars was lifted in two counties and from then on BB appeared in the official pedigree statistic (see table 1). But in 1963 the last pedigree herd was closed and the BB breed was considered as being extinct. Similarly to SH, however, one commercial breeder kept a non-pedigree herd and applied in 1987 for State support to maintain it as a genetic resource. His herd, of which not all animals had complete pedigrees, was blood typed in the Göttingen Laboratory and its genetic distance to the main West German contemporary breeds was calculated. Since no close relationship of these BB animals to any of the major breeds was found we encouraged the State to support it as genetic resource population. In 1988 the herd was registered with 4 boars and 23 sows in the Osnabrück Herdbook Society and purebred BB animals got 150 DM State subsidy. This made the BB attractive to more breeders, and by 1990 8 herds with 10 boars and 81 sows were registered. However, this subsidising scheme did not contribute much to the conservation of the breed. Within 3 years 2 of the original 6 sire families were lost while large numbers of progeny from the most frequent line were produced and sold to external customers who ate them. Consequently the subsidising scheme was changed and from 1993 on only 30 planned purebred litters and 10 selected boars were subsidised with yearly 500 DM each. This scared away two larger business-minded breeders but helped several hobby breeders to engage in the conservation project with different small families (see table 4) and to do good work until 1998.

Table 4. Number of State subsidised BB-breeding animals (M/F) and pedigree herds.

Year	Breeding herds*								AI-boars	Sum		
	a	b	c	d	e	f	g	others		herds	boars	sows
1988	2/13	3/15	2/13						-	3	7	41
1989	2/13	2/25	2/13						-	3	6	51
1990	2/14	2/35	2/12		0/2	0/5		3/3/13	1	8	10	81
1991-92	Subsidising scheme to 10 boars, 30 purebred litters											
1993	2/8	-	-	2/7	0/3	2/5	-	1/2/7	2	5	10	30
1994	2/7			2/8	1/3	2/5	1/4	1/0/3	1	6	10	30
1995	3/8			2/7	1/2	1/4	1/3	1/1/4	1	6	10	28
1996	3/8			2/8	1/3	1/3	2/5	1/0/3	1	6	10	30
1997	3/9			3/9	1/3	1/3	1/4	3/0/13	1	8	9	28
1998	3/9			3/8	1/3	1/2	-	2/1/4	-	6	10	26
1999	3/17			2/14	1/3	-	-	-	1	3	6	34
2000	3/17			3/14	-	-	-	-	-	2	7	31

*number boars/sows in herds a-g; no. herds/boars/sows in others.

Unfortunately in the two very bad pig years 1998 and 1999 five small herds in the conservation programme gave up, leaving only the two largest herds with 6 instead of the 10 required boars (plus one AI-boar), but they kept enough sows to get the 30 purebred litters. In the meantime in the EU-RESGEN project frozen semen of 22 BB-boars was collected which guaranteed the necessary population size until some new BB breeders from non herdbook herds claimed to be known to GEH may have been recruited.

In summary, the BB breed is a good example of the volatility of too small *in situ* conservation populations, and the essential role that parallel *in vitro* storage (here semen freezing) could play in such animal genetic resources maintenance programmes (Glodek, 2000).

Chapter 1.4. Pig genetic resources of Italy

G. Gandini[1], F. Fortina[2], O. Franci[3], G. Madonia[4] and D. Matassino[5,6]

[1]*Istituto di Zootecnica, Università di Milano, Via Celoria 10 - 20133 Milan, Italy*
[2]*Dipartimento di Scienze Zootecniche, Via Leonardo da Vinci 44 - 10095 Grugliasco, Italy*
[3]*Dipartimento di Scienze Zootecniche, Via delle Cascine 5 – 50144 Florence, Italy*
[4]*Istituto Sperimentale Zootecnico, Via Roccazzo 85 – 90136 Palermo, Italy*
[5]*Dipartimento di Scienze Zootecniche e Ispezione degli Alimenti – Via Università 100 – 80055 Portici, Italy*
[6]*Consorzio per la Sperimentazione Divulgazione e Applicazione di Biotecniche Innovative (ConSDABI), Italian National Focal Point - FAO, Azienda Casaldianni - 82020 Circello, Italy*

1. Changes in pig genetic resources during the last century

The panorama of pig genetic resources in Italy in the early decades of the last century included twenty-one local pig "breeds" (Table 1) and some additional varieties (Mascheroni, 1927). Many of these "breeds" where characterised by both high heterogeneity and high degree of similarity with other "breeds" and they should be considered as geographical varieties of a smaller number of distinct breeds. Nevertheless, at the beginning of the 20th century, Italy accounted for a relatively high pig diversity.

Table 1. Italian local pig "breeds" in early 1900, by region (see also text).
In bold, breeds which are still farmed today.

Region of farming	Breed - Population
Piemonte	*Cavour, Garlasco*
Lombardia	*Lombarda*
Emilia	*Reggiana, Modenese, Bolognese,* **Romagnola**
Veneto	*Friulana*
Toscana	**Cinta Senese**, *Cappuccia, Maremmana*
Umbria	*Perugina*
Marche	*Marchigiana*
Abruzzo	*Abruzzese*
Lazio	*Romana*
Campania	**Casertana**
Basilicata	*Cavallina*
Puglia	*Pugliese*
Calabria	**Calabrese**
Sicilia	**Siciliana or Nera Siciliana**
Sardegna	**Sarda**

Only five Italian local breeds are still farmed today, in most cases with a small number of sows. These are, from North to South, the *Mora Romagnola*, the *Cinta Senese*, the *Casertana*, the *Calabrese* and the *Nera Siciliana (*also called *Siciliana)* breeds, and are described in 3. In addition, a highly heterogeneous local pig population is still present in Sardinia, which frequently interbreed with both wild boars and commercial breeds.

The decline of local breeds is the result of a series of factors that arose with the intensification and industrialisation of pig farming, especially for production of the traditional dry ham, the modification in land use and the importation and diffusion of foreign high productive breeds. The first recorded importation, within this process, is that of *Yorkshire* boars in 1873, followed by other British and North American breeds. With respect to Northern Italy, where extensive farming with local breeds started to disappear early last century, Italian pig breeds showed in Southern and Central Italy a slightly higher resistance to the diffusion of commercial breeds. In 1950 the *Yorkshire* breed already represented more then 50%, 45% and 30% of pig herds farmed in Northern, Central and Southern Italy respectively (Feroci, 1979). In the second half of the last century the process of decline highly accelerated, leading most of local pig breeds to lose their individual identities and finally to extinction.

Most of the local Italian pigs are thought to belong to the same Iberian group as those in South of Spain, Portugal and France or, alternatively, to be intermediate between European and Indochinese pigs (Porter, 1993). The current EU Pig biodiversity project should provide elements to better investigate into these two theories.

2. Management of pig genetic resources in Italy

An official herdbook for swine breeds was established in Italy based on directive 88/661/CEE as implemented at the national level by law 30/91. The National Pig Breeder Association (ANAS) was put in charge for keeping the herdbook and for organising pig breeding schemes. Herdbooks did exist before 1991, based on private initiatives and under the control of the Ministry of Agriculture. Concerning local breeds, an herdbook for the *Cinta Senese* breed was active between 1934 and 1968, then re-opened in 1997. Finally, the new national law 280/99 gave a new definition for pig herdbooks (recording animals undergoing the same breeding schemes) and Pig Pedigree Registry (recording animals for the purpose of breed preservation) and put in charge ANAS for keeping them. An updated version of the disciplinary for the Pig Pedigree Registry is under approval, that will include all five Italian local breeds, *Cinta Senese*, *Mora Romagnola*, *Casertana*, *Calabrese* and *Siciliana*.

The main goals of the Pig Pedigree Registry are:
a) to collect pedigree information on animals corresponding to breed standards;
b) to implement policies aimed to the preservation of endangered breeds.

The Pig Pedigree Registry acts with the support of several research institutions by means of local offices based at the local breeder associations in most Italian provinces.

Although CEE Regulation 2078/92 did not consider endangered pig breeds as being eligible for economic incentives, the Tuscany Region has for the last twenty years been providing incentive payments to the farmers of the *Cinta Senese* breed in order to compensate for the lower profitability of the local breed compared to more profitable commercial breeds. The recent CEE Regulation 1257/99 will include the pig species in the payment schemes for endangered local breeds.

3. The Italian pig local breeds

There are five Italian local pig breeds which are still farmed today and which have been recently included in the Pig Pedigree Registry:
- *Calabrese* (CA: see plate 14);
- *Casertana* (CT: see plate 15);
- *Cinta Senese* (CS: see plate 16);
- *Mora Romagnola* (MR: see plate 17);
- *Nera Siciliana* or *Siciliana* (NS: see plate 18).

These five breeds have been all considered in the RESGEN12 project. Information on these breeds are available in both EAAP and FAO animal genetic resources data banks (see appendix to chapter 1.1).

3.1. Calabrese breed (CA)

Origin and distribution
The presence in the Calabria region of the *Calabrese* pig is documented at least from late 19th century. Its origins are unknown, but it was probably related to other black populations farmed in Southern Italy, now extinct, in particular with the *Pugliese* which was farmed in the bordering Apulian region. Four local varieties could be identified in the first half of the last century (Giuliani, 1940): *Reggitana*, *Cosentina*, *Catanzarese* and *Lagonegrese*. Immigration from several commercial breeds might have occurred in the last decades.

Breeding population numbers
There were about 150,000 heads in the 1940s, then the breed declined almost to extinction. In the late 1980s, E.S.A.C., the regional institution for agricultural development, identified and collected in its experimental farm at Acri, near the city of Cosenza, the last remaining animals, about 12 sows and 6 boars, which are the founders of the current population. Today there are about 65 sows in two conservation herds (at the centres ConSDABI and ARSSA). A few small herds and isolated animals are bred in the Pollino, Sila and Aspromonte mountains, in the Calabria and Basilicata regions.

Breed description
The head is rather long with a straight profile. The ears are relatively short and grow with a forward slant. The limbs are strong and long, but with poor hams. Skin and coat colours are black. Height at withers is about 0.75 m.

Qualification of breed
This pig was known to have a high degree of rusticity and hardiness and to be well adapted to free-range pasture in woods and fields. Growth performances were not evaluated in the RESGEN12 project because they were already object of investigation at ConSDABI, near Benevento. In the past the breed was accounted for a good precocity and prolificacy. When slaughtered between 16 and 18 months of age, it weighted from 140 to 180 kg.

Conservation issues
This breed has lost its bond with the area in which it was traditionally farmed. Today it is found only in a conservation herd in Calabria, in the Centre of ARSSA at Acri, and in a herd outside its original farming area, at ConSDABI. Conservation priorities in the short term include:

- to increase the number of sows and boars (*i.e.* the population effective number) in order to control genetic drift and inbreeding. This might be done both by increasing the size of conservation herds and by giving animals to those local farmers that show interest to raise again the breed;
- to register all animals in the Pig Pedigree Registry;
- to set up a genetic management scheme that will include all herds;
- to include the breed in the semen bank. Semen should be stored as back up in case of breed extinction as well as to be used in a cryo-aided live conservation scheme to minimise genetic drift;

- to link again the breed to some of its typical meat products, which are now made with meat from the large commercial breeds.

3.2. Casertana breed (CT)

Origin and distribution
The *Casertana* is an old breed, known at least since the end of the 18th century. Many theories are given about its origin and most agree that it received Asian blood at some stage. The breed takes its name from the city of Caserta. However, by the end of the 19th century it had a much wider distribution, including the entire Campania region as well as parts of the bordering northern regions of Lazio and Molise. Synonyms for the *Casertana* are *Napolitana*, *Teano* and *Pelatella*, which means bald. This breed is most probably the descendant of the Neapolitan breed imported into United Kingdom in late 18th to improve the old English types, in particular the *Berkshire*. Two varieties were recognised in the 20th century, that differed mainly in size.

Breeding population numbers
There were about 200,000 heads in the early fifties. Contrary to other local breeds, the breed was rarely crossed with the *Large White* because the presence of white and hairless patches in the F1 crosses was not compatible with sun exposition in the outdoor rearing. Nevertheless, the breed declined almost to extinction because it could not compete with the improved breeds in terms of prolificacy and lean cuts composition. Today there are about 28 sows at the ConSDABI conservation farm and additionally 15-20 sows in small herds.

Breed description
The conical head is rather long, with a wrinkled face and a straight profile; the small ears growth forward and there are often two wattles hanging down behind the jaw. The skin is slate-black all over, without bristles, except for little black hair on the head, neck and legs. The back is slightly arched, the rump is sloping, the legs are slender.

Qualification of breed
Growth performances were not evaluated by RESGEN12 because they were already object of investigation at ConSDABI Institute. In the recent past the breed was accounted for good precocity and low prolificacy. In adults, weight at withers is 55-65, body length 90-120 cm. When slaughtered at 12 months of age, it weighted from 150 to 250 kg with a good dressing percentage (85%). The breed was adapted both to grazing and fattening under intensive conditions. The quality of its fat was particularly appreciated.

Conservation issues
The *Casertana* is still farmed in a limited area, near the town of Benevento. A conservation herd is kept at ConSDABI. As for the *Calabrese* breed, conservation priorities in the short term include:
- to increase the number of sows and boars (*i.e.* the population effective number) in order to control genetic drift and inbreeding. This might be done both by increasing number and size of conservation herds and by giving animals to those local farmers that show interest to raise again the breed. A project to distribute boars to farmers started in 1999.
- to register all animals in the Pig Pedigree Registry;
- to set up a genetic management scheme that will include all herds;

- to enlarge the semen bank started within the RESGEN12 project. Semen should be stored as back up in case of breed extinction as well as to be used in a cryo-aided live conservation scheme to minimise genetic drift;
- to link again the breed to some of its typical meat products, which are now made with meat from the large commercial breeds.

3.3. Cinta Senese breed (CS)

Origin and distribution
This breed, well characterised by a white belt around the fore part of the black body, is thought to originate in the Montagnola uplands near Siena, in Tuscany (Dondi, 1924). Then it spread into other areas of Tuscany where it replaced smaller primitive local populations. Several old paintings testimony the presence of belted pigs in Tuscany since 14th century. In the last decades the *Cinta Senese* has been crossed with the *Large White* to produce an F1 hybrids, known as Siena Grey pigs (local names are *bigio* or *trimacchiato*).

Breeding population numbers
In 1934 the herd-book and the control of performances were started. In the early fifties there were about 160,000 heads. Nevertheless, because the changes in agriculture systems, the breed started to decline and reached the number of 90 sows in the eighties. Today there are about 200 sows in 50 herds, descending from 29 founders. Only three, among the 30 current herds, have more than 10 years of activities; most of farms begun to raise this breed very recently, often for hobby reasons or as part of tourism enterprises.

Breed description
The head has medium length with a straight profile. Ears are relatively large and point forwards and slight downwards. The body is cylindrical with robust limbs. The white belt (skin and hairs) is around the fore part of the body and includes withers, shoulders and forelegs. The black areas of the body have black skin with short, fine hairs. F1 crosses with *Large White* boars are well characterised by a white coat with two large slate-grey patches on the neck and the loin-rump regions.

Qualification of breed
This breed has a high degree of rusticity and it is well adapted to oak and chestnut wood pasture. Adaptation to free-ranging farming is maintained in crosses with *Large White*, but it is lost in backcrosses with the commercial breed (75% of *Large White* genes). Similarly to the other local breeds, it is a rather late maturing pig. The breed reaches the weight of 140 kg. in ten-eleven months at station. In the traditional extensive conditions, depending upon food availability, it takes fifteen or more months to reach 140 kg.. Dressing percentage is 81% with 58% of lean cuts.

Conservation issues
The *Cinta Senese* breed experienced a severe bottleneck in the 1980s. In the 1990s, population size increased, however uncontrolled breeding resulted into unbalanced founder contributions and high mean relationship. For these reasons, in the last twenty years inbreeding rapidly increased to the current level of 0.17. A management scheme to reduce inbreeding in the short term was recently developed (Gandini *et al.,* 2000). Following this scheme, females and males of nucleus herds are selected by minimising relationship; after selection (table 2), mean relationships among females, males, and between females and males can be reduced respectively by 40%, 25% and 43%, the effective number of founders

increased by 48%. The effective population size is 47, corresponding to an expected inbreeding rate per generation of 0.01. By assigning specific boars to each female herd, mean mating relationship can be further reduced. We are now implementing this scheme.

Table 2. Mean kinship and effective number of founders in the Cinta Senese breed, before (first row) and after (second row) selection.

Kinship among females	Kinship among males	Kinship between females and males	Number of founders	Effective number of founders
.270	.275	.261	29	9.5
.162	.206	.149	29	14.1

Besides inbreeding control, several actions have been taken to increase the value of the breed, including:
- the evaluation of a dry ham made with *Cinta Senese* pigs and with its crosses with the *Large White*;
- the request of Guarantee of Origins Protection (DOP; Regulations CEE 2081/92) for the *Cinta Senese* meat;
- research on extensive and semi-extensive farming systems, considering also crosses with the *Large White* (see plate 19). The use, in crossing, of the improved breed as paternal line should help in maintaining a viable population of the local breed.

3.4. Mora Romagnola breed (MR)

Origin and distribution
According to the prevailing theories, the origin of this breed goes back to the Iberian type. Three local varieties (*Forlivese*, *Faentina* and *Riminese*) were identified in the late 19th century (Tonini, 1949), when the *Mora* was farmed in the Eastern Emilia Romagna plain and on the Appennini mountains. The breed was officially named *Mora* in 1942. It was also known as *Castagnona* or *Bolognese*. No information are available on immigration from other breeds. In the first half of the last century, it was largely used to produce F1 crosses with the *Large White*.

Breeding population numbers
More than 22,000 heads were bred in 1920, and about 7,500 in 1953. The breed was nearly extinct in 1982 (two boars and two sows only survived in one farm, near Faenza). In the last two years the number of the *Mora* pigs increased: today there are 57 sows and 23 boars distributed in 15 herds. Many of these animals are kept for hobby reasons outside the region of origin. Control of performance and pedigree registration started respectively in 1999 and 2000.

Breed description
Breed standards were proposed in 2000 by the Breeders Association: long and dipping back body; long head with slightly convex profile; tapering snout covered by forward growing ears; dark grey or black upper-side skin, pink underside skin; dark brown bristles with coppering hue; ridge of thicker bristles along the back; long tail. Pigs have reddish hairs until two months of age.

Qualification of breed
Growth performances are under investigation at the University of Turin. When pigs are properly fed slaughtering weight (170 – 180 kg) can be reached in 18 – 20 months. Dressing percentage is about 80%. Young animals are well adapted to grazing, but fattening should occur under intensive conditions.

Conservation issues
The current *Mora Romagnola* population descends from four founder animals, two sows and two boars. Because of this tight bottleneck, the average relationship among the animals is extremely high and the question is raised on whether the breed still retains enough genetic variation for its survival and development. The number of herds increased from one to sixteen in the last three years and a Company working in pig meat transformation has recently shown interest to rescue the breed and to use purebred animals and crosses. A research project has just started, which aims to evaluate meat quality of *Mora Romagnola* pigs slaughtered at 150-160 kg for the typical "Culatello" ham.

3.5. Nera Siciliana or Siciliana breed (NS)

Origin and distribution
The *Nera Siciliana* of today derives from a population whose presence in Sicily is documented at least from the 19th century. The *Casertana* breed has been often said to have influenced this population. Several varieties were described in the past, including the most reported *Calascibetta* variety. More recently and until ten years ago, two populations were recognised, the *Madonie* and the *Nebrodi* pigs. Today the *Nera Siciliana*, also called *Siciliana*, is only found in the area of the Nebrodi mountains, in North-Eastern Sicily. In the last century, the original Sicilian pig population of Iberian type has been influenced in some areas from some crossing with improved breeds. However, most of the current *Nera Siciliana* population does not show evidence of crossbreeding.

Breeding population numbers
Accurate censuses of the *Nera Siciliana* are difficult because this breed is farmed on a large mountainous area, often in small numbers in a subsistence economy and no animal or farm registration exists. The 1998 census (Madonia *et al.,* in prep.) indicated a population of about 600 sows distributed in 130 herds. In addition there is a free-ranging populations of almost 200 sows. Comparisons with previous census estimates suggest that the *Nera Siciliana* breed is declining.

Breed description
The head is long with a straight profile. The ears point forwards and slight downwards. There are often two wattles hanging down behind the jaw. The body is short with long and robust limbs but poor hams. The size is relatively small, but with a certain variation among animals. Skin and coat are black. Twenty percent of the animals has small white markings on their face and fifteen percent has a white belt around the thorax. White marks over the legs are sometimes observed. Often there are bristles forming a ridge along the back and neck.

Qualification of breed
A late maturing pig, reaching 100 kg under semi-intensive conditions in twelve months and under the free-ranging traditional system at nineteen months of age. Dressing percentage is 82% with a percentage of lean cuts of 55%. Animals are slaughtered at winter for the local market. Precocity is good. This breed is characterised by a very high rusticity and hardiness.

Most of sows are mated to boars which are free-ranging all year around in harsh mountain areas that in winter can be covered by snow.

Conservation issues
This breed, for some aspects together with the *Cinta Senese* pig, is, among the five Italian local pig breeds, the only one which is still deeply rooted into the traditional farming system and which plays a certain economic role in its farming area. The *Nera Siciliana* breed is today declining, population size is probably below 900 sows, but there are still conditions for developing successful *in situ* conservation programmes.

Within the RESGEN12 project several actions were taken:
- to resume the traditional salami of S.Angelo di Brolo and to link it to the *Nera Siciliana*, which is its original breed. Salami were prepared following the traditional recipes and matured in both a controlled and traditional environment. Preliminary actions were taken for the request of the Guarantee of Origins Protection (DOP; Regulations CEE 2081/92);
- to create a niche market for the meat of the *Nera Siciliana*;
- to improve the traditional farming system techniques, in order to reduce age at slaughter.

Among others, the following initiatives should also be taken:
- to start registration in the Pig Pedigree Registry, but avoiding the risk of penalising the free-ranging farming system were the most typical animals are found;
- to discourage uncontrolled crossbreeding with improved breeds.

Acknowledgements

This work was financed by CE Regulation 1467/94, Contract RESGEN12. The authors are grateful to ANAS, APA of Siena, APA of Ravenna, ARSSA and ARAS for providing information.

Chapter 1.5. Pig genetic resources of Spain

J.V. Delgado[1], C. Barba[1], J.R.B. Sereno[1], A. Poto[2], A.M. Martínez[1], J.L. Vega-Pla[7], L. Sánchez[3], M.R. Fresno[4], A. Cabello[5] and M. Gómez[6]

[1]*Unidad de Veterinaria. Departamento de Genética. Universidad de Córdoba. (Spain)*
[2]*Centro de Investigación y Desarrollo Agroalimentario. Murcia. (Spain)*
[3]*Departamento de Producción Animal. Facultad de Veterinaria. Lugo. (Spain)*
[4]*Instituto Canario de Investigaciones Agrarias. Tenerife. (Spain)*
[5]*Centro de investigación y desarrollo Agrario. Exsma. Diputación Provincial de Córdoba (Spain)*
[6]*Diputación Foral de Bizkaia. Servicio de Ganadería. Bilbao. (Spain)*
[7]*Laboratorio de Grupos Sanguíneos. Cría Caballar. Córdoba (Spain)*

1. Introduction

Spain is populated by pig breeds classified into three different ethnic types (Delgado *et al.*, 2000a). Located in the north-west of the Iberian Peninsula, the Celtic breed arrived with the civilisations which invaded this area from central and northern Europe. These pig resources are specialised in meat production but they do not present the capacity for the fat infiltration into the muscle fibre.

The second type was the Mediterranean pig breed which arrived in Spain with the civilisations which invaded the Iberian Peninsula from the Mediterranean Basin, populating the south-east of the Iberian Peninsula and the Balearic Islands. Most of the breeds currently included within this type present a tendency for fat infiltration into the muscle fibre.

The third type, found only in the Canary Islands, originated from north west Africa, where religious beliefs have resulted in the extinction of most of the region's pig breeds.

In the past, there was a rich diversity of pig breeds in Spain, particularly within the Celtic and Mediterranean varieties, which were widely distributed and numerous. These local breeds were raised in large herds under extensive conditions, or in family herds bred in groups of no more than eight to ten, for the family's own use.

At the beginning of the 20th century, six pig breeds were classified within the Spanish Celtic Type. The most important of these were the *Celta Gallego* (Galizian Celtic: see plate 20) and the *Chato Vitoriano* (Vitorian flat-nosed), which counted thousands of breeding females. Other minor breeds of this type should also be mentioned: *Asturiano* breed (Asturian pig), perhaps an "intermediate" between the Celtic and Mediterranean branches; *Vich* or *Catalan* breed(Catalonian); *Lermeña* breed from Burgos and *Baztanes* breed from Navarra.

The Mediterranean type was represented by the complex Iberian branch which populated the majority of "Dry Spain". This branch demonstrated a special genetic diversity showing several strains and ecological adaptations, such as the *Retinto Extremeño* (Iberian red: see plate 26) and the *Negro Lampiño* (Iberian Black, hairless: see plate 24). Older varieties include the *Mamellado* (Wattles) and *Dorado Gaditano* (Cadiz Golden) while other modern varieties such as *Villalon, Retinto Portugués, Torbiscal, Entrepelado* and *Silvela* should also be mentioned.

Differentiated breeds within the Mediterranean type include the *Porc Negre Mallorqui* (Black Mallorcan: see plate 25) and the *Vasco* (Basque pig) and also modern breeds like the *Manchado de Jabugo* (Jabugo Spotted: see plate 22) and the *Chato Murciano* (Murciano flat-nosed: see plate 21), derived from the Iberian type by crossbreeding with foreign breeds at the beginning of the 20th century.

The *Negro Canario* (Black Canarian Pig: see plate 23) is the only representative of the African pig of the Canary Islands. Around 1954 traditional management systems began to be replaced by a new intensive system based on the breeding of selected foreign breeds imported from central Europe and the British Isles (Rodero *et al.,* 1994). By the eighties, most of the breeds mentioned previously were either extinct or close to extinction.

The state of the Celtic type was critical, only the highly endangered *Celta Gallego* remained. Certain strains of the Mediterranean type became extinct but in general this type was more fortunate. The *Vasco* breed has disappeared in Spain, but some stock is being introduced from France. Although well established, the Iberian pig suffers from a lack of internal genetic diversity, because most production has been concentrated in only four varieties (*Retinto Extremeño, Entrepelado, Torbiscal and Negro Iberico*). As a result, the remaining varieties are close to extinction or have disappeared, as in the case of the *Dorado Gaditano*.

The previously endangered *Porc Negre Mallorqui* (Payeras, 1998) is now increasing in number in response to the conservation programme developed in the Balearic Islands (Jaume *et al.,* 1997). Active programmes of conservation are also in place for the endangered *Manchado de Jabugo* (Barba *et al.,* 1999) and *Chato Murciano* (Poto *et al.,* 2000) breeds, which offer some hope for the future.

The *Negro Canario* was near extinction by the end of the eighties, but responded very well to conservation programmes during the nineties. Numbers are now sufficient to ensure its conservation (Robert *et al.,* 1998).

In Table 1 we present a summary of the current situation of all the breeds mentioned above. In this chapter, we will describe their present situation and the action developed for their conservation and preservation, using the experience of all the Spanish collaborators in the EU project RESGEN12.

2. What are we doing in pig conservation in Spain?

At this point we wish to describe the different activities developed in our country for the conservation of the native breeds of pig. Some are linked to the objectives defined in the EU project RESGEN12, but others are complementary to these.

2.1. Primary characterisation

Using the network structure of the Spanish Society for the Conservation of Domestic Animal Genetic Resources (SERGA) we have collected and permanently updated the information regarding the present situation of our native pig breeds, taking into account data about the population structure, animal characteristics, production and management systems. This information is enclosed in the FAO databank, the EAAP databank, and the national databank (see URLs in the Appendix to chapter 1.1).

2.2. Morphological characterisation

Negro Canario was the first Spanish native pig breed whose morphotype was determined statistically (López *et al.,* 1992). Recently an intensive study of the Iberian pig has been undertaken to compare qualitative and quantitative traits among its varieties, in order to characterise the entire breed in all its diversity (Pardo *et al.,* 1998; Mata *et al.,* 1998; Delgado *et al.,* 1998 and Delgado *et al.,* 2000b), a study which has also included the *Manchado de Jabugo* as well as the *Chato Murciano* (Poto *et al.,* 2000). The other breeds are in the process of morphological characterisation.

Table 1. Situation of pig genetic resources in Spain (in bold: breeds included in the RESGEN12 project).

Breed	FAO Risk status[1]	Population trend	Conservation programme
Celta type			
Celta Gallego	Endangered	Increasing	Yes
Chato Vitoriano	Extinct	-	-
Asturiano	Extinct	-	-
Vich or Catalan	Extinct	-	-
Lermeño	Extinct	-	-
Baztanes	Extinct	-	-
Mediterranean type			
Retinto Extremeño*	Not at risk	Increasing	Yes
Negro Iberico*	Endangered	Decreasing	Yes
Silvela*	Not at risk	Decreasing	Yes
Villalon*	Endangered	Decreasing	Yes
Dorado Gaditano*	Extinct	-	-
Mamellado*	Endangered	Decreasing	Yes
Torbiscal*	Not at risk	Increasing	Yes
Retinto Portugués*	Endangered	Stable	Yes
Entrepelado*	Not at risk	Increasing	Yes
Negre Mallorqui	Endangered	Increasing	Yes
Vasco	Critical	Stable	-
Chato Murciano	Critical	Increasing	Yes
Manchado de Jabugo	Critical	Decreasing	Yes
African type			
Negro canario	Endangered	Increasing	Yes

[1] as defined in table 2 of chapter 1.1.
*Breeds belonging to the Iberian branch.

2.3. Genetic characterisation

Through national initiatives all varieties of the Iberian pig and the *Manchado de Jabugo* have been characterised and more recently the *Chato Murciano*, using the panel of 27 microsatellites recommended by the ISAG /FAO advisory group for animal genetic distance work. Nei (1972) and Reynolds (1983) genetic distances among these populations are presented in Table 2. Those results have been discussed in detail by Martinez *et al.* (1998a, 2000a, 2000b and 2000c) and the conclusions will only be briefly summarised here. A clear divergence was shown among the *Duroc*, *Chato Murciano* and the Iberian pig group, but no clear differences could be established among the Iberian varieties, except *Negro Lampiño*, *Torbiscal* and *Manchado de Jabugo* (sometimes considered as a different breed). The traditional grouping of Iberian varieties around 3 types, red, black and spotted, appeared to be not entirely supported because the *Entrepelado* variety, usually considered as a member of the black group, was in fact closer to the red varieties *Retinto Extremeño* and *Silvela*. Also *Torbiscal*, though showing red colours, was well differentiated from the *Retinto Extremeño* group and from *Negro Lampiño*. It is also worth noting that the *Chato Murciano* breed appeared to be less related to the Iberian varieties (distance ranges 0.30-0.40 and 0.52-0.70 in Table 2) than to the *Duroc* (0.26 and 0.43). This may be a consequence of the conservation programme recently implemented for extending the genetic basis of the breed (as described below).

The incidence of the halothane gene in the *Manchado de Jabugo* (Ramos *et al.*, 1999) has also been estimated. The Iberian pig varieties *Retinto* (*Extremeno*) and *Negro Iberico* (*Lampino*), together with *Manchado de Jabugo* and *Negro Canario*, were tested for biochemical polymorphisms comparatively to other European breeds in the RESGEN project, and for microsatellites in the pig genetic diversity study called PIGBIODIV (see table 3 of chapter 3.1).

Table 2. Pairwise genetic distances between Iberian pig varieties, Chato Murciano and Duroc, calculated using Reynolds (above the diagonal) and Nei standard (below the diagonal) distances.

	RP	MA	EN	RE	NI	TO	SI	MJ	DG	CM	DU
RP	*****	0.1842	0.0930	0.1102	0.1552	0.1817	0.1059	0.2697	0.1703	0.3194	0.2177
MA	0.3385	*****	0.0838	0.0962	0.1659	0.1752	0.0971	0.2303	0.1607	0.3325	0.2419
EN	0.1676	0.1740	*****	0.0274	0.1009	0.1466	0.0306	0.1975	0.0724	0.3000	0.1710
RE	0.1886	0.1887	0.606	*****	0.0914	0.1673	0.0316	0.2027	0.0910	0.3182	0.1946
NI	0.2677	0.3118	0.1775	0.1582	*****	0.1395	0.0745	0.2587	0.1041	0.3177	0.1892
TO	0.3020	0.3040	0.2546	0.2836	0.2328	*****	0.0931	0.2764	0.2017	0.3848	0.2769
SI	0.2252	0.2319	0.0945	0.0948	0.1811	0.1980	*****	0.1893	0.0816	0.2962	0.1727
MJ	0.3589	0.3057	0.2688	0.2646	0.3639	0.3773	0.2968	*****	0.1089	0.4021	0.3236
DG	0.3144	0.3217	0.1597	0.1875	0.2081	0.3650	0.2107	0.4745	*****	0.3238	0.1612
CM	0.5173	0.5607	0.5230	0.5395	0.5451	0.7033	0.5950	0.6002	0.5507	*****	0.2616
DU	0.4274	0.5230	0.3390	0.3809	0.3693	0.5733	0.3947	0.5144	0.3348	0.4328	*****

Breed/variety code: RP: Retinto Portugués, MA: Mamellado, EN: Entrepelado, RE: Retinto Extremeño, NI: Negro Iberico (Lampiño), SI: Silvela, TO: Torbiscal, MJ: Manchado de Jabugo, DG: Dorado Gaditano, CM: Chato Murciano, DU: Duroc.

2.4. Productive characterisation

Iberian pig performances have been studied intensively. Three phases of the productive life of these animals were investigated, taking into account pre-weaning, post-weaning and post-mortem characteristics (Barba, 1999).Similar studies were developed of the *Manchado de Jabugo* but including only the first two phases (Forero, 1999 and Forero *et al.*, 1999).

In other breeds such as *Negre Mallorqui*, *Celta Gallego* and *Chato Murciano* productive studies are in progress. Reproductive performance has been studied in the Iberian pig and *Manchado de Jabugo* (Suarez *et al.*, 1999) as well as *Negre Mallorquí* (Jaume *et al.*, 1999).

2.5. Creation of gene banks

Recently the Spanish government has regulated the organisation of domestic animal gene banks, creating a duplicated structure with a central institution located in CENSYRA, Colmenar Viejo (Madrid), which is in charge of the national bank, and a network of regional banks located in autonomous regions.

Presently our team features two active laboratories for collection, processing and conservation of pig germplasm. One is located in CIDA, Murcia, and the second at the University of Cordoba. Our activities have focussed on two points, the first was methodological, applying the new technique of Thilmant (1997) to our native breeds. After some modifications this technique has offered great results which duplicate the efficacy of the conserved doses with respect to our traditional technique (Westendorf, 1975), including post-freezing fertilisation (Poto *et al.*, 2000).

The second was the creation and development of the Iberian pig, *Manchado de Jabugo* and *Chato Murciano* germplasm bank (see chapter 4.2 of this book).

2.6. Creation of protected quality marks for products

The introduction of officially-regulated protected quality marks for pig products certifying origin, defining the breed, animal management system and meat processing system has played an important role in the protection of the Spanish native pig breed. In this area, the Iberian pig is the most advanced with at least four marks (Extremadura, Jabugo, Guijuelo and Valle de los Pedroches). Also important is the development of a protected mark for the *Negre Mallorqui* traditional meat product "sobrasada" (Jaume, 1999).

A protected quality mark for a *Celta Gallego* dry meat product "lacon gallego", has produced a very good result.

There is still a lot to be done in this area, particularly in those breeds which as yet do not have this protection, because we have noted spectacular results in the increase of outputs, census and herd number of those breeds featuring this quality mark measure.

3. Conservation programmes for the Spanish native pig breeds

3.1. Celta Gallego

This breed was very close to extinction in the eighties, but the work undertaken in the nineties by a group of conservationists led by Dr Luciano Sánchez established the first stages of a conservation programme for this breed. Their activities were primarily directed towards the organisation of the breeders creating the specific Association. Secondly they established a recuperation programme supporting the *Bísaro* Portuguese breed, a related breed also belonging to the Celtic type.

After the increase in census of breeding females to over 100 they have worked hard to promote these pigs' natural products, such as a dry ham known as "lacon gallego". They have increased the profitability of this pig, especially those fattened with chestnuts, the traditional feeding system.

Today this breed is expanding and the creation of a gene bank is planned. Some Galician researchers have been trained in implementing the Thilmant (1997) method of semen freezing by one of us (A.. Poto) within the activities developed in the EU project RESGEN12.

3.2. Iberian pig

In 1996 we started work on the EU Project RESGEN12 whose objectives featured two of the most important varieties of the Iberian pig, *Retinto* and *Negro Iberico*, but soon we noted, as stated earlier, that the problem in the Iberian pig was not so much the loss of a breed as the lack of genetic diversity within a branch.

Traditionally the existence of several varieties within the Iberian pig breed is well known These varieties corresponded to several levels of subdivision, from strains to old varieties and ecological differentiations, but they were not generally well defined or characterised.

Coinciding with our work in RESGEN12, in 1996 we designed an ambitious project whose main objective was a clear definition of the population structure of the Iberian pig studying the different varieties existing today. The work was planned in four stages:
- Primary characterisation and databank;
- Morphological characterisation (quantitative and qualitative traits);
- Productive characterisation (pre-weaning, post-weaning and slaughtering traits);
- Genetic characterisation (Microsatellites and Halothane or RYR1 locus).

The participants in this project are the Spanish Ministry of Agriculture, the association of breeders (AECERIBER), the Centre of Selection and Reproduction of Badajoz (CENSYRA), the provincial governments of Cordoba and Huelva and the Department of Genetics at the University of Cordoba.

With the support of RESGEN12 and other national resources, in 1997 we started developing a gene bank of the Iberian pig. In this way we created a station for the collection, processing and cryoconservation of semen with 12 stables (boars), and began the activities. Today we have worked with 18 Iberian boars. Soon the same work will be started in Extremadura by the CENSYRA of Badajoz. The result of the investigation and development of these projects will be presented in chapter 4.2 of this book

As regards *in situ* conservation, we have to draw attention to the work developed by the provincial governments of Cordoba and Huelva, and the government of Extremadura, which have established policies of cession of animals belonging to different varieties of the Iberian pig to farmers. The varieties to be mentioned are *Torbiscal* (Huelva and Cordoba), *Silvela* (Huelva), *Negro Ibérico* (Huelva) and *Retinto Extremeño* (Extremadura). Each year thousands of animals belonging to the afore-mentioned varieties are distributed to farmers.

3.3. Manchado de Jabugo

This breed has been included in the programme described for the Iberian pig varieties regarding characterisation. Additionally the Provincial Government of Huelva maintains two conservation herds with ten females and four boars in each one of these herds.

From this flock each year is establish a campaign of cession to farmers of the province.

Five males of these breed have been submitted to semen collection in the University of Cordoba, as will be pointed out in chapter 4.2. In the near future other sets of animals of the breed will be added to the genebank.

3.4. Chato Murciano

This breed is relatively young, since it was created at the beginning the 20th century by crossbreeding native females of the Mediterranean type with some foreign breed boars (Large White and Berkshire among others). The breed expanded quickly thorough the Murcia Region until the census in the fifties was over a thousand. In the seventies the breed went into dramatic crisis until the mid-nineties when the government of Murcia introduced a programme of conservation.

At the start of the programme there were only 23 purebred animals(8 boars and 15 sows), which moreover presented a suspected high level of inbreeding. For this reason the researchers planned the conservation and extension of the genetic basis simultaneously, by using a stock of 23 females crossbred at different levels. The mating scheme included using backcrosses with purebred boars grading in order to increase the census as quickly as possible Today there are around sixty breeding females pure or graded up to at least the fifth generation.

The breed has been characterised from the morphological and productive point of view as will be shown in sections II of this book. The breed has also been genetically characterised as shown above (see table 2).

This breed has the largest gene bank of the Spanish breeds (see chapter 4.2).

3.5. Negre Mallorqui

The establishment of the herdbook in 1997 was the first initiative in the conservation plan of the Negre Malloqui. This was supported by the creation of a specific breeders association. Alongside these two measures the Balearic government launched an initiative to promote this animal's traditional products, "sobrasada" and "porcella". These products have now obtained the trademark IGP from the EU.

The Association conducts a disease control programme including a permanent veterinary assistance. Also data on reproductive performances of the female have been recorded, which will be presented in chapter 2.4.

We have to point out some preliminary studies of genetic characterisation using biochemical polymorphisms (Albumin, Pre-Albumin, Transferrins and Post-Albumin), and eight microsatellites among those proposed by the ISAG/FAO Committee mentioned before. So genetic characterisation of this breed has started, however without yet allowing an evaluation of its genetic distance with respect other

3.6. Euzkal Txerria

The *Euzkal Txerria* pig became extinct in Spain in the eighties, but some farmers of the Basque country started a breed expansion programme using animals from France, where this breed is well maintained (see chapter 1.2). Today these animals have not yet been introduced.

3.7. Negro Canario

When the Spanish conquerors reached the Canaries in the 15th century they found a pig breed distributed throughout the seven islands of this archipelago. There is evidence that animals belonging to this breed were carried on Columbus' first trips to America (Rodero *et al.,* 1992). After the conquest and over the centuries, this animal was practically the only pig breed present in the Canaries, but with a slight influence of other foreign breeds such as Iberian, British breeds, etc. The white pig industry nearly drove the *Negro Canario* to extinction, when its size went down to only 30 breeding females.

During last years, the governments of La Palma, Tenerife and later on Gran Canaria started programmes of conservation, but these were not well co-ordinated. Nevertheless these programmes successfully incorporated other islands (La Gomera, Lanzarote) into this action, and increased the census up to a present number of 240 sows.

The breed was morphologically characterised by López *et al.* (1992), but no studies on genetic and productive characterisation have been carried out. This breed was included in the genetic distancing programme of the RESGEN12 project (see section III of this book).

Some animals of this breed have been recently relocated to the Centre of Agricultural Investigation and Development (CIDA) of Murcia (South-east Spain), for collection and freezing of semen, but no results have yet been obtained.

At least four programmes of cession of animals to farmers exist in order to increase population size and to reintroduce these animals to the Canaries. In the near future, efforts will be directed towards the constitution of a regional breeders association to avoid the present uncoordinated actions among the different islands.

SECTION II

BREED EVALUATIONS (PERFORMANCES)

Chapter 2.1. Performances of French local breeds

F. Labroue[1], H. Marsac[1], M. Luquet[1], J. Gruand[2], J. Mourot[3], V. Neelz[4], C. Legault[5] and L. Ollivier[5]

[1]*I.T.P., Pôle Amélioration de l'Animal, BP 3, 35651 Le Rheu Cedex, France*
[2]*I.N.R.A., Station Expérimentale de Sélection Porcine, 86480 Rouillé, France*
[3]*I.N.R.A., Unité Mixte de Recherche Veau Porc, 35590 Saint-Gilles, France*
[4]*C.T.S.C.C.V., 7 avenue du Général de Gaulle, 94704 Maisons-Alfort Cedex, France*
[5]*I.N.R.A., Station de Génétique Quantitative et Appliquée, 78352 Jouy-en-Josas Cedex, France*

1. Reproduction traits routinely recorded

The performance traits routinely recorded concern litter size (numbers of total born, live born and weaned piglets). However, the total born is sometimes not available, so only live born and weaned piglets have been analysed (Marsac *et al.,* 1999 ; Labroue *et al., 2000b*).

The evolution of the number of litters recorded per breed over the 5 past years is given in table 1. For 4 breeds, the total number of litters increased regularly. The most important increase was observed for the *Gascon* (+ 81%), and then for *Limousin* (76%), *Basque* (70%) and *Bayeux* (57%). As for the *Blanc de l'Ouest*, the number of litters increased until 1998, but started decreasing in 1999. One explanation may be the practice of crossbreeding with selected lines, which leads to less purebred litters in that breed. The classification between breeds is the same as for the number of sows: *Gascon, Basque, Limousin, Blanc de l'Ouest* and *Bayeux* (see table 1 of chapter 1.2). However, the average number of litters per sow per year is very low, often below 1 litter per sow per year on average.

The evolution of the number of live born piglets per breed over the 5 past years is also given in table 1. In 1999, the best results appeared in *Gascon* and the worst in *Bayeux*. However, the range between breeds is narrow, around 7.5 - 8 live born piglets per litter. Whatever the breed, the number of live born piglets tended to decrease over the 5 past years. One possible explanation of this phenomenon is the increasing number of litters declared to ITP. As a matter of fact, results of the earlier years, which included smaller numbers of litters, might have excluded lower litter sizes and led to an over estimation.

The evolution of the number of weaned piglets per breed over the 5 past years is given in table 1. In 1999, *Gascon* had the best results with nearly 7 weaned piglets per litter, *Blanc de l'Ouest* and *Bayeux* were very close to each other (between 6 and 6.5 weaned piglets) and the worst results were seen in *Basque* and *Limousin*, with less than 6 weaned piglets per litter. So, despite similar numbers of live born piglets, the number of weaned piglets clearly differed from one breed to another. These results highlight the best breeding conditions and/or maternal abilities of *Gascon* sows (higher number of functional teats in particular) and, to a lesser extent, of *Blanc de l'Ouest* and *Bayeux*.

To sum up, the study of reproduction traits in the 5 French local breeds highlights several weaknesses such as the very low number of litters per sow per year. Such a trait could be improved through better management during both the mating and farrowing periods. In the same way, it should be possible to improve the number of weaned piglets per litter by a simple selection based on teat number. In addition, litter size should also increase if the mean age of breeding sows decreased, for example by practising an earlier culling of sows, which presently occurs around the 7th parity.

Table 1. Reproduction traits per breed and per year.

Breed	Traits	1995	1996	1997	1998	1999
Basque	litters recorded	82	120	174	191	277
	live born piglets	8.3	8.6	8.4	8.1	7.7
	weaned piglets	6.5	6.7	6.5	6.0	5.5
Blanc de l'Ouest	litters recorded	45	50	54	88	72
	live born piglets	9.0	9.4	8.1	8.0	7.4
	weaned piglets	7.9	8.0	6.9	6.4	6.5
Bayeux	litters recorded	21	30	29	35	49
	live born piglets	7.0	6.5	6.4	7.9	7.3
	weaned piglets	6.0	5.4	5.4	5.8	6.2
Gascon	litters recorded	59	89	129	230	306
	live born piglets	8.5	8.0	8.4	8.0	8.1
	weaned piglets	6.8	6.9	6.9	6.8	6.9
Limousin	litters recorded	24	20	74	72	101
	live born piglets	7.6	8.6	7.0	6.7	7.4
	weaned piglets	6.5	6.3	5.2	5.3	5.8

2. Production traits

Because production traits are not routinely recorded on farms, they have been studied in an experimental farm (Goumy, 1999; Labroue *et al.*, 2000a). Results are only available for 4 local breeds because the size of the *Bayeux* breed was not large enough to provide 48 piglets. The aim of the present study is to compare growth, carcass and meat quality traits of four different local breeds of pigs (*Gascon, Basque, Limousin* and *Blanc de l'Ouest*) with a *Large White* control. This comparison was made under two different finishing conditions - semi-confined *vs.* extensive - and for two slaughter weights (100 *vs.* 150 kg).

2.1. Experimental protocol

A total of 48 piglets per breed entered the INRA-SESP experimental station of Rouillé (Vienne), at a liveweight of 25 kg, in order to be tested between 30 and 100 kg liveweight (Goumy, 1999). For each breed, animals came from at least 12 different litters, in order to be representative of the breed, and the balance between females and castrated males was respected.

The birth dates were planned in order to make it possible for all genetic types to reach the live weight of 100 kg over a short period of time. After fattening, one third of the pigs were slaughtered at 100 kg. The others were dispatched into two kind of finishing conditions - semi-confined or extensive - and slaughtered at about 150 kg. The breakdown of slaughtered animals by breed and by treatment is given in table 2.

The *Large White* control makes it possible to connect the different genetic types, in particular between slaughter batches, because it was impossible to have all local breeds represented in each slaughter batch. For that purpose, the total number of *Large White* pigs put into test (easily available) was twice as large as in the other breeds. However, only 41 *Large White* pigs were taken into account in the analysis.

Table 2. Breakdown of slaughtered animals by breed and by treatment.

Breed	Slaughter at 100 kg	Slaughter at 150 kg		Total
		Semi-confined finishing	Extensive finishing	
Basque	12	16	15	43
Blanc de l'Ouest	15	9	16	40
Gascon	8	16	18	42
Limousin	12	12	13	37
Large White	16	15	10	41
Total	63	68	72	203

2.2. Traits recorded on farm

Growth, feed efficiency and fatness performances are given in table 3. Between 30 and 90 kg liveweight, the ranking of breeds was the following: *Large White, Blanc de l'Ouest, Limousin, Gascon* and *Basque*. Between 100 and 150 kg liveweight, the ranking was the same whatever the finishing conditions: *Large White, Blanc de l'Ouest, Gascon, Limousin* and *Basque*. Growth rate was lower after 100 kg than before for all genetic types. In addition, differences between breeds appeared to be smaller during the finishing period, because only the *Large White* significantly differed from local breeds. Lastly, the slowing down of growth during the finishing period was lower in *Gascon* and *Large White* than in the other breeds.

Table 3. Growth, food efficiency and fatness traits (least squares means).

	Basque	Gascon	Limousin	Blanc de l'Ouest	Large White
Average daily gain $_{30-90}$ (g)	560 a	563 a	633 b	682 c	848 d
Average daily gain $_{100-150}$ (g)	316 a	362 a	337 a	374 a	542 b
Average daily gain $_{30-150}$ (g)	443 a	455 a	476 ab	504 b	671 c
Feed conversion ratio	3.93 a	3.84 ab	3.73 b	3.16 c	2.55 d
Backfat thickness $_{90\ kg}$ (mm)	32 a	33 a	41 b	23 c	13 d

On the same line, values with no letter in common are significantly different (P< 0.05).

The feed conversion ratio between 30 and 90 kg liveweight, estimated per pen, was lower for *Large White* than for local breeds, which thus showed a better food efficiency. *Blanc de l'Ouest* was intermediate between *Large White* and the 3 other local breeds. *Basque* and *Gascon* had the highest feed conversion ratios. The classification between breeds was exactly the opposite of that observed for average daily gain during the same period.

2.3. Carcass traits recorded in abattoirs

Carcass results are given in table 4 for both slaughter weights (100 and 150 kg). Compared with *Large White* control, local breeds appeared much fatter whatever the slaughter weight (higher fat thickness, lower percentage of ham and loin, higher ratio of loin over back fat). This situation results from the lack of selection in local breeds, except for *Blanc de l'Ouest*, the closest breed to *Large White*. *Blanc de l'Ouest* has indeed benefited from breeding programmes until the middle of the 1970s.

Table 4. Carcass and meat quality traits (least squares means).

Trait	Basque	Gascon	Limousin	Blanc de l'Ouest	Large White
Slaughter at 100 kg					
Slaughter weight (kg)	105 ab	100 a	106 ab	109 b	107 ab
Dressing percentage (%)	72.9 a	70.6 a	72.4 a	74.8 a	72.7 a
Carcass length (mm)	948 a	927 a	875 b	1009 c	990 c
Fat thickness (mm)	41 a	44 a	51 b	29 c	20 d
% Ham + Loin	52 a	51 ab	49 b	56 c	62 d
Loin / Back fat ratio	1.76 a	1.12 b	1.28 b	2.42 c	4.54 d
ultimate pH GS	5.69 ab	5.85 a	5.83 a	5.65 b	5.57 b
water holding score GS	11.4 a	8.2 ab	5.4 b	9.7 ab	12.8 a
L* GS	51 ab	49 ab	48 a	50 ab	51 b
a* GS	10.1 a	11.1 a	9.8 a	9.1 a	6.1 b
Slaughter at 150 kg					
Slaughter weight(kg)	154 a	146 b	142 b	147 ab	149 ab
Dressing percentage (%)	73.2 ab	74.4 a	73.5 ab	72.9 ab	72.1 b
Carcass length (mm)	1044 abc	1027 ab	966 b	1123 c	1092 ac
Fat thickness (mm)	48 a	49 a	56 b	32 c	23 d
% Ham + Loin	53 a	52 a	52 a	58 b	62 c
Loin / Back Fat ratio	1.53 a	1.27 a	1.15 a	2.28 b	3.77 c
pH at 45 minutes LD	6.27 a	6.41 b	6.27 a	6.02 c	6.42 b
ultimate pH SM	5.86 a	5.87 a	5.96 a	5.81 a	5.65 b
water holding score LD	9.1 a	10.5 a	8.9 a	10.1 a	14.3 b
L* LD	47 a	46 a	47 a	47 a	50 b
a* LD	10.9 a	10.1 a	9.5 ab	8.0 b	5.8 c

On the same line: values with no letter in common are significantly different ($P < 0.05$). GS = Gluteus superficialis; LD = longissimus dorsi; SM = semi membranosus. L* = brightness value; a* = red saturation value.

Limousin was characterised by the highest fatness. *Basque* and *Gascon* were intermediate between *Blanc de l'Ouest* and *Limousin*. Both *Large White* and *Blanc de l'Ouest* had the significantly longest carcass at 100 kg whereas *Limousin* had the shortest. At 150 kg, the same classification between breeds remains, however the differences were not significant.

Lower dressing percentages were always observed in *Large White*, although no significant effect of breed was evidenced.

2.4. Meat quality traits and halothane sensitivity

Meat quality traits (pH, water holding capacity and colour measurements) comparisons are also given in table 4. The lowest pH45 (pH at 45 minutes *post mortem*) were observed for *Bayeux*, *Blanc de l'Ouest* and *Limousin*. This trait being strongly related to stress level before slaughter, that means that some local breeds may be more sensitive to transportation stress than improved breeds such as the *Large White*. In addition to their lower pH45, local breeds also presented a lower water holding capacity, though the differences were significant only at 150 kg slaughter weight. In contrast, the ultimate pH was higher in the local breeds compared to the *Large White* control, though not all differences were significant at 150 kg slaughter weight. The ranking among the 5 breeds for ultimate pH was exactly the same as for fatness. For colour measurements, *Large White* is characterised by a lighter meat colour (higher brightness values of L*) with less saturated red (lower values of a* for similar values of b*).

The darker meat colour for local breeds primarily comes from the higher ultimate pH values. High pH is indeed responsible for the oxidation of myoglobin, the main meat pigment.

The meat quality results of table 4 may also be discussed in relation to the possible existence of carriers of the gene for halothane sensitivity in some local breeds. A sample of each French local breed was typed for the RYR (ryanodine receptor) locus of halothane sensitivity. A large variation was found in the frequency of the halothane-sensitive allele, which went from zero in *Basque* (on 48 pigs) to 44 % in *Bayeux* (on 96 pigs), with low values in *Gascon* (1 % on 42 pigs) and *Limousin* (5 % on 68 pigs) and an intermediate value of 34 % in *Blanc de l'Ouest* (on 135 pigs). This investigation indicates some introgression of the halothane gene from *Piétrain* or similar breeds into several local breeds. Among the 4 local breeds compared, the *Blanc de l'Ouest* breed showed the lowest values in all 3 pH results of table 4, which might be partially explained by the high frequency of the halothane gene in this breed. The *Blanc de l'Ouest* situation probably reflects the history of the breed mentioned in chapter 1.2, and particularly the introduction of *Veredeltes Landschwein* in the late 1960s. Similar explanations may also account for the *Bayeux* situation. Crosses between *Piétrain* and *Bayeux* have indeed been reported in the past (Quittet and Zert, 1971), though it is difficult to assess the respective parts played by these distant crosses and more recent ones with *Blanc de l'Ouest*.

2.5. Biochemical analysis

Biochemical analysis (total lipids percentage and fatty acids composition) were performed on a sample of *Longissimus dorsi* and a sample of back fat. Results are given in table 5.

Table 5. Biochemical analysis (least squares means).

	Basque	Gascon	Limousin	Blanc de l'Ouest	Large White
lipids in back fat (%)	83 a	82 a	81 a	76 b	72 b
intra-muscular fat (%)	3.9 a	3.2 b	3.4 ab	2.9 b	1.9 c
Fatty acids composition in backfat:					
saturated fatty acids (%)	43.1 a	46.6 b	46.3 b	41.3 c	41.7 c
mono-unsaturated fatty acids (%)	45.2 a	43.5 b	43.9 b	46.8 a	42.4 c
poly-unsaturated fatty acids (%)	11.7 a	9.9 b	9.9 b	12.0 a	16.0 c

On the same line. values with no letter in common are significantly different (P< 0.05).

Lipid percentage in both muscle and back fat was strongly related to carcass fatness. *Large White* differed from local breeds by lower lipid levels (for both lipids in back fat and intra-muscular fat). Lipid percentage in back fat was higher for local breeds than for control, although *Blanc de l'Ouest*, the leanest genetic type among local breeds, did not significantly differ from *Large White*. This higher lipid percentage in back fat led to a better cohesiveness of fatty tissues, which is a necessary quality for the process of meat products such as dried sausages.

Concerning the fatty acid composition in back fat, *Large White* and *Blanc de l'Ouest* had the lowest percentage of saturated fatty acids. So the back fat of local breeds, with high unsaturated fatty acids contents, yielded a more wholesome food from a nutritional point of view. Unsaturated fatty acids led however to softer fat, because their melting point is lower than for saturated fatty acids. They are also more sensitive to oxidation, which might cause conservation problems.

2.6. Sensory analysis

The sensory analysis of roasts included an evaluation by consumers and an evaluation by expert referees. The results are given in table 6.

Table 6. Sensory analysis: evaluation by consumers and expert evaluation.

	Basque	Gascon	Limousin	Blanc de l'Ouest	Large White
Evaluation by consumers (82 adults)					
Score of global acceptability (scale 0-10)	6.4 a	6.2 a	6.4 a	6.4 a	3.7 b
Positive intentions of re-consuming (%)	73.2	64.6	78.1	70.7	23.2
Negative intentions of re-consuming (%)	26.8	35.4	21.9	29.3	76.8
Intentions of re-consuming (Chi-square test result)	yes	yes	yes	yes	no
Expert evaluation[1] (13 referees x 4 replications)					
Slice aspect:					
loin eye area / total meat area (%)	9.1 b	8.8 b	9.0 b	9.5 a	9.7 a
fat area / total slice area (%)	1.6 b	2.2 a	2.2 a	1.2 c	0.9c
Flavour:					
metallic flavour	0.6 b	0.9 b	0.7 b	1.3 a	1.4 a
fat flavour	1.7 a	2.0 a	2.0 a	1.3 b	1.1 b
Texture:					
firm texture	4.7 c	5.0 c	5.4 c	6.3 b	7.1 a
dry texture	4.4 b	4.7 b	4.6 b	6.0 a	6.5 a
juicy texture	2.9 ab	3.4 a	3.3 a	2.4 bc	2.1 c
fat texture	1.9 a	2.3 a	2.2 a	1.4 b	0.9 c

[1]For means of scores (scale 0-10), on the same line, values with no letter in common are significantly different (P< 0.05).

The local breeds roasts were significantly preferred to *Large White* roasts, according to the note of global acceptability. Positive intentions of re-consuming were in a range of 65 % for *Gascon* to 78 % for *Limousin*, versus only 23 % for *Large White*.

Large White roasts significantly differed from local breeds roasts by 2 criteria: firmer and less fat texture. These two characteristics seemed to explain why consumers rejected *Large White* roasts. The firmer and less fat texture of *Large White* roasts might have originated in the lower intra-muscular fat percentage.

For several criteria, *Large White* significantly differed from 3 local breeds (*Basque, Gascon, Limousin*) but not from *Blanc de l'Ouest*. The characteristics of these three local breeds were the following:
- lower loin eye-area relative to the total meat area,
- higher fat area relative to the total slice area,
- less pronounced metallic flavour,
- more pronounced fat flavour,
- less dry and juicier texture.

The lower loin eye area as well as the higher fat area for these three local breeds could be related to their higher carcass fatness. The texture criteria could be related to both water holding capacity and intra-muscular fat, which stimulates salivary secretion. So, the higher intra-muscular fat percentage of the three local breeds led to a juicier and less dry texture of the meat, despite the lower water holding capacity. In our study, the differences of meat flavour only appeared between *Gascon* on one hand and *Large White* and *Blanc de l'Ouest* on the other hand, *Basque* and *Limousin* being intermediate.

3. Conclusions

To sum up, the results confirmed the low performances of local breeds compared to *Large White* for average daily gain, feed efficiency and carcass lean content. Local breeds were also characterised by their higher dressing percentage and higher ultimate pH, which could probably be related to carcass fatness. They also showed a darker meat colour, due to the higher ultimate pH. On the contrary, local breeds had a lower pH 45, which means they were probably more sensitive to pre-slaughter stress, such as transportation, than the *Large White* control. Biochemical analysis performed on pigs slaughtered at 100 kg showed higher intra-muscular lipid level for local breeds in comparison with the controls. The sensory evaluation by experts revealed the fatter and less firm texture of roasts from local breeds, which could explain their being preferred by consumers. The forthcoming results of processing and sensory quality of dry-salted hams will complete this study and will make it possible to establish the effects of breeding conditions and/or breed on both meat processing traits and quality of final product.

Due to their generally lower level of performances, economic benefits from local breeds cannot be derived from the usual trading channels. In contrast, owing to their higher meat quality, these breeds appear to be well adapted to the processing of top quality products. The examples of both *Basque* and *Gascon* and to a lesser extent of *Bayeux* illustrate that genetic conservation can be compatible with economic sustainability. As regards the *Blanc de l'Ouest* and *Limousin*, the most likely use will be in crossbreeding with maternal selected lines, especially in the framework of new quality labels such as the «label rouge» and/or organic production. In that case however, the genetic management will have to be controlled in order to avoid the total extinction of the original pure breeds.

Chapter 2.2. Performances of German local breeds

P. Glodek[1], W. Chainetr[1], M. Henning[2], E. Kallweit[2] and K. Fischer[3]

[1]*Institute for Animal Breeding and Genetics, University of Göttingen, Albrecht-Thaer-Weg 5, 37075 Göttingen, Germany*
[2]*Institut für Tierzucht und Tierverhalten, FAL Mariensee, 31535 Neustadt, Germany*
[3]*Institut für Fleischerzeugung, BAFF, E.-C.-Baumann-Strasse 20, 95236 Kulmbach, Germany*

1. Purebred dam systems

Since German Saddlebacks (*Angler Sattelschwein* (AS), *Deutsches Sattelschwein*(DS), *Schwäbisch-Hällisches Schwein*(SH)) as well as *Bunte Bentheimer* (BB) are registered in herdbook organisations they undergo routine litter recording and are also allowed to send sib groups to test stations for fattening and carcass evaluation. While the former is obligatory for all sows in herdbook farms, the latter is regularly utilised by active boar breeders only. Station tests are used by Saddleback breeders only occasionally and they have not been used at all by BB-breeders for more than 10 years. In the following section, the routine information collected and published in ZDS (Zentralverband der Deutschen Schweineproduktion) annual reports (the latest came out 1999 and contained data of 1998) will be given. Additionally, results from an experiment in which the LWK (Landwirtschaftskammer) Hannover compared samples of AS, SH, BB with pure *Piétrain* (PI) and two *Piétrain* crosses at a test station will be presented.

1.1. Reproductive performances

In table 1 recent results of litter recording are given for 1998. AS and DS are considered as one breed in the ZDS-statistics and for BB the last three years are summarised.

Table 1. Litter recording performances of Saddleback and BB sows in comparison with the standard dam German Landrace (DL) in 1998 (ZDS, 1999).

Trait	AS/DS	SH	BB*	DL (Standard)
No. sows recorded	230	135	103	36031
No. litters per sow and year	2.0	2.1	1.9	2.2
No. born alive/litter	11.0	10.8	10.3	10.3
No. weaned/litter	10.0	9.4	9.3	9.5
No. born alive/sow and year	22.3	22.4	19.1	22.5
No. weaned/sow and year	20.1	9.6	17.4	20.7
Rearing losses (%)	9.9	12.5	8.8	7.9

*litter records of 1996,1997 and 1998 combined.

The figures show that all three resource breeds (particularly BB) were kept under less intensive production conditions than the DL-standard dam breed, and that therefore their performance per sow and year was lower and the rearing losses were higher than in DL. But in litter size all three resource breeds competed favourably with DL, so they seemed to have retained their originally good reproductive performance (see also table 2 in chapter 1.3).

1.2. Fattening carcass and meat quality traits

In table 2 available station test results from the last two ZDS annual reports are summarised, for male castrates and females separately in the testing period 30-105 kg liveweight.

Table 2. Fattening and carcass performances of Saddleback pigs (1997 and 1998 combined) in comparison with DL standard pigs (ZDS, 1999).

Trait	AS/DS		SH	PI x SH	DL (standard)	
	M	F	M	F	M	F
No. pigs tested	15	25	45	142	4 988	460
Daily gain (g)	808	720	810	836	893	955
Feed conversion ratio(kg)	3.22	3.19	2.87	3.02	2.72	2.63
Carcass length (cm)	98.60	99.60	99.40	95.80	102	101
Backfat thickness (mm)	35	33	35	25	26	25
Loin eye area (cm^2)	31.60	36.80	36.30	55.60	44.30	46.40
Lean-fat-area ratio (fat/lean)	0.89	0.73	0.68	0.29	0.51	0.37
pH (45 min. *post. mortem*)	6.25	6.42	6.45	5.99	6.46	6.43
Meat colour (Opto-Star: higher score for darker meat)	61.9	68.90	70.50	62.40	73	69

M = castrated males, F = females.

The figures must be interpreted with caution because they represent raw means over different stations with different breed sampling and management standards, only feed composition and measuring techniques were the same. It can be seen that both Saddleback populations had lower growth rate and poorer feed efficiency, which to a great deal resulted from their considerably higher fat content (lean-fat ratio and backfat thickness) and much smaller loin-eye areas. But it can also be seen that *Piétrain* x SH crossbred females are leaner than DL females but do not reach their growth rates and feed efficiency, which is explained by 749 g daily gain and 60.5 cm^2 loin eye area of purebred *Piétrain* females in 1998 over all stations. In meat quality traits, only *Piétrain* x SH crossbreds were as expected inferior to all other breed groups which reached high quality standards.

In 1996 the LWK Hannover (Schön and Brade, 1996) ran a test of so called "old breeds" at its Station Katlenburg, in which small samples of all three breeds AS, SH, BB were compared with purebred *Piétrain* (PI) and single crosses PI x AS, PI x SH and DE x DL male castrates as another control. The data were analysed separately for castrated males (fed restricted after 60 kg) and females fed ad libitum (see table 3).

PI-purebreds were in both sexes the leanest pigs with the poorest meat quality and by far the lowest daily feed intake. But the slowest growing and least efficient purebreds were in both sexes BB, which also produced the fattest barrows and second fattest gilts, however, they had larger loin eyes than AS females and SH males.

Table 3. Fattening, carcass and meat quality traits of "old" breeds and their PI crosses as compared to sire (PI) and dam (DE x DL) breeds standards (Schön and Brade, 1996).

Traits	Females					Castrated males						
	PI	AS	BB	PIxAS	PIxSH	PI	AS	SH	BB	PIxAS	PIxSH	DExDL
No. pigs tested	43	12	21	15	78	15	15	74	19	17	70	89
Daily gain (g)	694	778	635	800	723	768	843	706	683	814	756	852
Feed conversion ratio	2.82	3.01	3.19	2.70	2.75	2.74	2.94	3.19	3.30	2.88	2.86	2.76
Feed intake (kg/day)	1.95	2.35	2.03	2.15	1.97	2.00	2.44	2.22	2.21	2.32	2.14	2.32
Carcass length (cm)	94.60	98.10	96.60	97.30	97.80	94.80	99.10	101.50	96.10	96.80	94.40	100.90
Backfat thickness (mm)	18	32	29	28	23	24	32	32	32	33	27	25
Loin eye area (cm^2)	63.50	43.60	48.30	51.50	55.20	57.50	43.90	38.40	42.30	46.70	50.90	46.70
Lean-fat area ratio (fat/lean)	0.17	0.58	0.51	0.42	0.28	0.30	0.57	0.62	0.65	0.54	0.37	0.43
BF-Lean (%)*	65.70	54.30	56.10	58.40	61.70	61.70	54.00	53.10	52.60	55.10	58.70	57.20
Lean score belly (1 - 9)	7.60	3.30	2.80	4.10	6.30	4.80	2.70	3.00	1.90	2.90	4.60	3.90
pH (45 min)	5.53	6.25	6.11	6.10	5.93	5.61	6.06	6.32	6.14	6.09	5.87	6.12
Meat colour (Opto-Star: higher score for darker meat)	64.00	70.90	72.50	67.50	69.90	67.00	68.80	72.00	70.30	69.70	65.70	69.70
LF (24h)	8.56	3.61	4.91	5.41	7.27	8.40	5.26	3.28	4.47	5.81	7.46	5.12

*Lean content according to the Bonn formula, generally used in German test stations; LF (24h) = conductibility 24h *post mortem*.

The small sample of AS had by far the highest daily feed intake and growth rate among all purebreds in both sexes. Also PI x AS crosses were much better than PI x SH crosses in these traits. But the latter were distinctly better in lean content and gave in both sex-feeding regimes the second best carcasses of all groups. Apparently good selected PI-boars were used in the Schwäbisch-Hall region, where this is a popular market cross.

In meat quality traits the purebred PI pigs were distinctly the poorest, followed by the PI-crosses, particularly PI x SH which had the highest loin eye and lean content of all crosses. SH females and AS castrates had the best meat quality but BB purebreds showed the best meat colour although their pH(45 min *post-mortem*) was surprisingly low. This and their high loin eye seem to support rumours, that some *Piétrain* genes might have gone into BB earlier. This is also supported by results of the MHS-test (halothane gene) made in the purebred pigs by the LWK. The frequencies of the susceptibility gene P were found to be 100% in PI, 40% in BB and 20 % in AS, whereas SH had no P gene.

2. Crossbred dam systems

The purebred dam data have clearly shown that all three resource populations can only compete with the standard dam line DL in litter size. But neither in fattening nor in carcass quality traits can they compete even with DL, not to mention good crossbreds or modern hybrids. However, table 3 showed that well marketable products were obtained in single crosses of SH sows with selected PI-boars in the SH region. This cross was the basis of the "Bäuerliche Erzeugergemeinschaft Schwäbisch Hall (BEGSH)" set up in 1988, integrating 240 small farmers with more than 3000 producing sows in 1997. All crossbreds are slaughtered at one abattoir and marketed by BEGSH as brand name quality pigs in the region (Bühler, 1997). In addition the SH sows are also advertised as particularly suited to small ecologically producing farms thereby occupying another consumer favoured niche.

In larger intensively (or even outdoor) producing farms, however, a crossbred sow is also needed that falls not too far behind modern hybrid sows. It was therefore interesting to test whether such sows could be produced from crosses of gene resource local breeds and current white dam line breeds such as *Landrace* or *Large White*. If such sows were mated to current sire line boars even better final products could be expected compared to the single crosses in table 3, because they would have only 25 % of genes from the resource breeds.

2.1 Litter performances

In order to obtain results within the RESGEN period, we used semen of the first six boars in the freezing programme to produce crossbred litters from BHZP hybrid sows (*Large White* x *Landrace*) at our Relliehausen experimental farm and integrated 20 crossbred sows of each cross (DS- and BB-sire) into our production herd of BHZP type hybrid sows, used as control. Management of sow mating and culling was the same for all sows and all were routinely mated to the same two boar types: PI purebred and PI x *Hampshire* criss-crosses, both with normal halothane (NN) genotype.

The litter records are presented in table 4.

Table 4. Litter performances of DS-, BB-crossbred and hybrid control sows (Least squares means and significance; Chainetr, 2001).

Traits	DS	BB	Control	Total & Mean	Residual stand. dev.
No. litters	91	93	294	478	
No. pigs born alive	9.91 A	8.79 B	10.20 A	9.86	2.80
No. pigs weaned	8.18 ab	7.70 b	8.36 a	8.21	2.77
Mean birth weight (kg)	1.62 b	1.69 a	1.63 ab	1.64	0.25
Mean weaning weight (kg)	7.61 ab	7.71 a	7.31 b	7.44	1.50

Least-squares model: D (dam-), S (sire-breed), D x S Interaction, Parity (1-4), Season (1-7);
Significance level: A, B = P<.01; a, b = P <.05.

Table 4 shows that DS crossbred sows were not significantly different from control sows whereas BB crossbred sows produced significantly smaller litters at birth (-1.42 piglets) and at weaning (-0.65 piglets), this leading to significantly higher individual piglet weights. These results must be interpreted with caution since they were based on less than 100 litters and the management conditions in the experimental farm were affected by reconstruction in the farrowing house. Nevertheless, at least the DS crossbred sows were quite competitive with modern hybrid sows and tended also to live longer than these. Whether the BB crosses could reach similar levels should be investigated in broader field conditions.

2.2. Fattening carcass and meat quality traits

Live and net daily gain as well as the carcass grading with FOM are given in table 5. Again the progeny of DS and control sows were at the same level but BB progeny had significantly lower growth rates. It is interesting that in the price relevant FOM lean content no significant differences between all three groups were found. This is confirmed by the lean-fat ratios, despite significantly larger loin eye areas in both experimental groups compared to the controls.

Meat quality traits in table 5 show that PSE relevant pH-values reached a high and non significantly different level in all three progeny groups. GÖFO and conductivity values 24h *post mortem* were very good in all three groups, although slightly significant differences were found. The greatest surprise, however, was that the intra-muscular fat content was highest in progeny of control sows, followed by BB- and with a highly significant difference from the DS progeny. This finding fits into the picture of water content and LF24, and may have a reason in the highest loin eye area of DS crossbreds.

In another sample of 16 progeny from each of the three crosses (8 castrated males and 8 gilts) a sensory test was made at the BAFF Kulmbach by Dr. Fischer with a taste panel of 6 trained experts. The relevant figures found in this test are presented in table 6.

The test day had a significant effect for all sensory scores and the test person effect was highly significant for the last three traits in table 6 but not for juiciness and tenderness. All other factors in the statistical model were not significant for any of the sensory traits except the abnormal sour taste score. For the latter all effects were statistically significant at the 5 % level but the taste person effect was significant at the 0.1 % level, thereby indicating that the definition seems to be vague.

Table 5. Fattening carcass and meat quality traits of progeny from DS-, BB- and control crossbred sows (Least-squares means and significance, Chainetr, 2001).

Trait	DS	BB	Control	Total & Mean	Residual stand.dev.
No. Progeny (in brackets for meat quality traits)	220 (217)	243 (231)	573 (189)	1036 (637)	
Live daily gain (g)	652 Ba	641 Bb	668 A	661	58
Carcass daily gain (g)	430 A	418 B	432 A	430	26
FOM lean percent	56.38	56.22	56.56	56.36	2.41
Carcass length (cm)	98.10 B	98.00 B	99.10 A	98.30	2.40
Backfat thickness (mm)	24.90 B	23.60 A	23.60 A	24.40	2.90
Loin eye area (cm²)	50.64 A	49.81 Ab	47.84 B	49.41	4.13
Lean-fat-area ratio (fat/lean)	0.36	0.36	0.35	0.37	0.07
pH(45 min)	6.26	6.23	6.25	6.25	0.22
pH(24h)	5.42	5.42	5.42	5.42	0.08
GÖFO Colour (24h)	59.10 ab	58.80 b	59.70 a	59.20	3.00
LF (24h)	3.78 B	3.42 A	3.49 A	3.50	0.95
Intra-muscular fat (%)	1.69 B	1.87 A	1.91 A	1.82	0.62
Water content (%)	75.20 B	74.90 A	75.10 AB	75.10	0.70

Least-squares model: D (dam-), S(sire-breed), D x S Interaction, Sex, Season (1-11), Covariance (carcass weight);
Significance level: A, B = P<.01; a, b = P<.05;
LF defined in table 3.

Table 6. Sensory scores of progeny from DS -, BB-crossbred and hybrid control sows (Least square means and significance; Chainetr, 2001).

Trait	DS	BB	Control	Mean	Residual stand.dev.
Loin eye area (cm²)	50.62	49.90	47.74	49.52	5.12
FOM lean percent	57.07 a	54.80 b	56.98 a	56.26	3.09
Juiciness (1-6)	3.48	3.60	3.43	3.53	0.83
Tenderness (1-6)	3.70	3.76	3.52	3.65	0.97
Aroma (1-6)	3.79	3.60	3.55	3.58	0.85
General score (1-6)	3.66	3.60	3.45	3.52	0.83
Sour taste (1-3)	2.72 a	2.51 b	2.63 ab	2.66	0.54

Least-squares model: D (dam-), S(sire-breed), D x S-Interaction, Sex, Tester (1-6), Test day (1-5);
Significance level: a, b = P<.05.

Unfortunately these small samples were not fully representative of the three crosses in the whole experiment as can be seen from the FOM lean percentage given in the second row of table 6 in comparison with table 5. Here BB progeny were significantly fatter than the other two groups and this may have affected the sensory scores. In the most important scores, namely juiciness and tenderness, BB progeny were the best and the controls the poorest but these differences reached only significance levels between 10 and 20%. In the typical pig aroma DS-crosses scored better than the other groups and reached similar significance levels. But DS progeny showed a higher frequency of abnormal sour taste, 1.7% and 13% significant compared to BB- and control progeny, respectively.

The conclusion of this experiment is that terminal products from a DS grand-dam were comparable to standard hybrids in growth and carcass grading but showed slightly inferior meat quality as far as intra-muscular fat and water content of the meat was concerned. Their sensory qualities, however, were not significantly different from BB progeny, in the typical pig aroma they scored best. Progeny of BB grand-dams were significantly inferior in growth rate but were similarly graded at the market and showed intra-muscular fat comparable to the controls and the best subjective score for juiciness and tenderness. It could then be stated that from both DS and BB resource breeds terminal pigs with well marketable carcass and top meat qualities would be obtained and that a clear tendency to better sensory eating qualities, such as juiciness and tenderness, was found by an expert panel of BAFF.

In an overall economic judgement, including the litter performance of the dams, this experiment has shown that a system with DS crossbred sows and their progeny from current boar types is quite competitive compared to standard commercial hybrids on present markets. For BB crossbred sows this cannot be concluded, since they had significantly lower litter performance and their crossbred progeny grew significantly slower. Even with comparable carcass grading the overall economy of BB crossbred sows will therefore be significantly lower than that of DS crossbred and control sows. Since these results have been obtained under intensive management conditions at our experimental station, they should be verified by field experiments in outdoor and ecological farming systems to which the resource breeds DS and BB are expected to be better adapted.

Chapter 2.3. Performances of Italian local breeds

O. Franci[1], G. Gandini[2], G. Madonia[3], C. Pugliese[1], V. Chiofalo[4], R. Bozzi[1], A. Acciaioli[1], G. Campodoni[1] and F. Pizzi[5]

[1]*Dipartimento di Scienze Zootecniche, Via delle Cascine 5 – 50144 Florence, Italy*
[2]*Istituto di Zootecnia, Università di Milano, Via Celoria 10 - 20133 Milan, Italy*
[3]*Istituto Sperimentale Zootecnico, Via Roccazzo 85 – 90136 Palermo, Italy*
[4]*Istituto di Zootecnia, Università di Messina, Via S.Cecilia 30 – 98123 Messina, Italy*
[5]*IDVGA-CNR, Via Celoria, 10 – 20133 Milan, Italy*

1. Introduction

Of the numerous pig breeds and varieties farmed in Italy at the beginning of the last century, five survived the post-war industrialisation process of pig production and are still reared today. Only two breeds, the *Cinta Senese* and the *Nera Siciliana* (also named *Siciliana*), with respectively 200 and 800 sows, still have an active role in the economy, albeit in rather restricted areas. The number of sows from the other three breeds, *Mora Romagnola*, *Casertana* and *Calabrese* amounts to less than a hundred and there is no longer a bond with the area in which they were traditionally reared; most of the animals are now farmed for conservation reasons.

In the light of these statistics, we decided to focus on the *Cinta Senese* and *Nera Siciliana* breeds for our study on growth, carcass and meat quality traits. We believed that this study would aid the development of activities able to enhance the economic profitability of these two breeds and avert the threat of extinction. It is highly probable that proper evaluation of local breeds, which identifies their valuable characteristics, will improve their market value.

Few data were available on the performance of these breeds before the beginning of the project RESGEN12; performance of *Cinta Senese* crosses with *Large White* were evaluated at station (Franci *et al.*, 1994a; 1994b; 1995; 1996; 1997) and some carcass and meat quality parameters were studied in *Casertana* pigs (Colatruglio *et al.*, 1996; Girolami *et al.*, 1996; Grasso *et al.*, 1996).

Accurate breed evaluation requires an understanding of the interactions between different management systems and breed characteristics with trials at station or under controlled field conditions and under the traditional Mediterranean extensive system. Other important issues are: evaluation of crosses, comparison with a commercial breed of reference and economic assessment. We decided to give priority to those experimental hypotheses to estimate the performance of the breeds that might be significant for economic viability and conservation. With this objective in mind we developed the research:

- to analyse performance under current farming systems in order to identify their limits and weaknesses and to propose solutions for their improvement;
- to give priority to farming systems that facilitate breed survival, such as the use of the local breed as female population in crossbreeding. The use of females, as opposed to males, guarantees the maintenance of a large population of the local genotype;
- to assess performance in high input systems, but monitor performance in traditional low-input extensive systems too, often characterised by harsh environments which bring out the hardiness of the local breed;
- to examine the characteristics associated with the production of typical food products, as the link between a local breed and local products can increase the breed's economic profitability;

- to carry out as much of the research as possible in the area where the breed is reared, in partnership with local research Institutes and Universities. This will stimulate farmers' interest in their breeds and involve local administrations in the development of plans to enhance the economic viability of the breed and to support its farming.

To achieve this we studied:
- growth, carcass and meat quality parameters in *Cinta Senese* pigs and its crosses with *Large White* (Campodoni *et al.*, 1999), both at station and under the traditional extensive farming system;
- growth, carcass and meat quality parameters in *Cinta Senese* (Franci *et al.*, 2000) and *Large White* at station;
- quality of dry-salted ham from *Cinta Senese* pigs and its crosses with *Large White*;
- growth, carcass and meat quality parameters of *Nera Siciliana* pigs, both at station and in the extensive traditional farming system, considering a set of different ages and weights at slaughter;
- the effect of different methods of maturing salami from *Nera Siciliana*, which we developed on the basis of traditional local recipes;
- reproductive traits in all five Italian local pig breeds.

Only certain research studies and results are reported here because of lack of space.

2. Production traits in the *Cinta Senese* and *Nera Siciliana* breeds

2.1. *Cinta Senese* breed

Experimental procedure
Seven *Cinta Senese* and two *Large White* sows were mated to two *Cinta Senese* and three *Large White* boars to produce *Cinta Senese* (CS), *Large White* (LW) and *Large White* x *Cinta Senese* (LWxCS) progeny. These animals were reared intensively in pens (IN) and fed usual commercial mixtures (17.7 % of crude protein up to 120 days of age and 16.3% subsequently) given semi-ad libitum (max. 2.5 kg/d). Contemporarily, progeny from three *Cinta Senese* sows and two *Cinta Senese* boars were reared under the traditional extensive system (OUT), in oak and chestnut woods pasture with moderate feed supplementation during spring and summer (max. 1 kg/d of a commercial mixtures with 17.7% crude protein). Following the traditional sylvo-pastoral management system, all males and females were castrated. On overall, 29 CS-IN, 29 LWxCS-IN, 12 LW-IN and 17 CS-OUT animals were slaughtered when they reached the appropriate weight for medium/heavy pigs (130-160 kg). Slaughter of CS-OUT pigs occurred after autumnal wood pasture.

At slaughter, carcasses were dissected according to "Modena" system and lean cuts (ham+foot, shoulder+foot, loin and neck), fat cuts (backfat, jowl, belly and kidney fat) and bone cuts (head) were weighed. The *Longissimus lumborum* muscle (LL) was tested for: (i) pH_{45} and pH_{24}; (ii) colour (CIE L*, a*, b*); (iii) chemical composition (A.O.A.C., 1980); (iv) water loss determined by pressure on filter paper (Grau and Hamm, 1952) and by cooking in water bath; (v) shear force (Warner-Bratzler, Instron) on raw and cooked meat. Right ham was processed according to the production method of the Tuscany dry-cured ham and weight loss during the salting period (21 days) was recorded. Analyses of variance, by means of GLM procedure (SAS, 1996), were performed separately for the three genotypes reared in confined conditions (CS-IN, LWxCS-IN, LW-IN) and for the comparison between *Cinta Senese* pigs reared in confined and extensive conditions (CS-IN, CS-OUT).

Growth

Figure 1 reports body weight as function of age. The sigmoidal curve, which is expected when feed requirements are met, is observed only under intensive conditions and in particular for LW-IN and LWxCS-IN pigs. Early growth of CS-IN seems curbed. This breed reached the weight of 140 kg one hundred days later than LW-IN. LWxCS-IN showed intermediate performance between parental breeds, except for early stages when performance were similar to LW-IN. The extensive conditions, due to limited food availability during spring and summer, severely restrained growth in CS-OUT pigs. These animals showed a marked compensatory growth during the final stage in the autumnal wood pasture. Growth curves of these animals are similar to those reported for the Iberian pig under the extensive traditional system (Mayoral *et al.*, 1999).

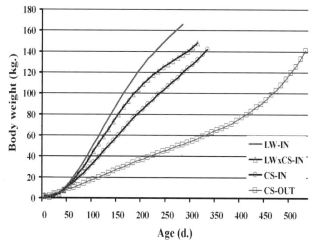

Figure 1. Growth pattern of Large White (LW-IN), Large White x Cinta Senese (LWxCS-IN) and Cinta Senese pigs (CS-IN) reared indoor and of Cinta Senese pigs (CS-OUT) reared under extensive conditions.

Comparison with Large White and crossbred under intensive conditions

Table 1 reports results for carcass traits. CS-IN pigs reached the target slaughter weight later than LWxCS-IN crosses and LW-IN pigs, respectively. In order to be slaughtered at an age suitable for heavy pig production (eight months), LW-IN animals reached a slaughter weight of 16-19 kg higher than CS-IN and LWxCS-IN pigs. CS-IN pigs showed lower dressing percentage and worse carcass traits (lower lean cuts percentage and higher fat cuts and bone cuts percentage) than the other two genotypes. For carcass composition, LWxCS-IN crosses showed somewhat intermediate values between the two pure breeds. Lower performance than in the commercial breed was expected in the *Cinta Senese*, as it has been observed in other local breeds, in particular under intensive production system. Daily gain of Iberian pigs was 2/3 of that of *Landrace* pigs and backfat thickness was twice as much (Serra *et al.*, 1998). In comparison with *Landrace* x *Large White* crosses, *Gascon* and *Limousin* breeds grew slower (537 and 600 *vs.* 811 g/d), had worse feed efficiency (4.5 and 4 *vs.* 3.2) and showed lower muscle percentage (39.6 and 38.4 *vs.* 52.8) (Legault *et al.*, 1996); *Basque*, *Gascon* and *Limousin* pigs grew 30% slower and produced 20% less of lean cuts than *Large White* pigs (Labroue *et al.*, 2000a).

69

Table 1. Slaughter traits of Cinta Senese, Large White and crossbred pigs reared indoors: means and residual standard deviation (r.s.d.).

	Genetic type			r.s.d.
	CS-IN	LWxCS	LW-IN	
Age d	312 a	273 b	259 c	15.60
Slaughter weight kg	136.00 a	138.90 a	154.70 b	6.88
Dressing %	81.18 a	83.07 b	82.79 b	1.78
Lean cuts %	57.69 a	62.70 b	69.12 c	1.85
Fat cuts %	36.77 a	31.90 b	24.76 c	2.00
Bone cuts %	5.14 a	4.81 b	4.93	0.40

Means with different letters differ at the 5% level.

The chemical-physical characteristics of LL are reported in table 2. The highest ultimate pH was in CS-IN and the lowest in LW-IN pigs. Serra *et al.* (1998) and Labroue *et al.* (2000a) found pH_{24} higher in local than in improved breeds (Iberian *vs. Landrace*; *Gascon, Basque, Limousin* and *Blanc de l'Ouest vs. Large White*, respectively). CS-IN and LWxCS-IN meat was more intensely coloured than LW-IN meat because of the greater red contribution. The lower hue values for CS-IN made meat from this local breed more acceptable than that of the crosses or of LW-IN pigs. Similar results, showing a local breed to have a better meat colour, were reported by Serra *et al.* (1998) on Iberian compared with *Landrace* pigs. The chemical composition data showed higher intra-muscular fat and lower moisture of CS-IN meat compared to LW-IN meat, with the crosses always somewhere in between, in line with the results obtained for other Mediterranean local breeds (Simon *et al.*, 1996; Serra *et al.*, 1998). It should be noted that the intra-muscular fat of CS-IN and of crossbreed pigs in this study falls within, or only slightly exceeds, the range (2-3 %) considered optimal for pork quality (Wood *et al.*, 1986; Bejerhom and Barton-Gade, 1986; Molénat *et al.*, 1992). CS-IN meat showed a better water holding capacity, evaluated either by pressure method or by cooked loss in LL muscle or as salting loss in the ham. Crossbreds were, as a rule, in an intermediate position with performances that were alternately more similar to that of the paternal or the maternal breed. Raw meat from CS-IN had higher shear force value than that of LW-IN, but differences disappeared after cooking.

Table 2. Meat quality traits of Cinta Senese, Large White and crossbred pigs reared indoor: means and r.s.d.

	Genetic type			r.s.d.
	CS-IN	LWxCS-IN	LW-IN	
pH$_{45}$	6.22	6.27	6.31	0.23
pH$_{24}$	5.78 a	5.67 b	5.50 c	0.19
Colour				
L*	49.66	51.55	51.44	4.20
chroma	12.35 a	12.46 a	10.23 b	2.01
hue	0.38 a	0.43 b	0.45 b	0.08
On wet basis %				
moisture	73.23 a	73.93 b	74.25 b	0.85
protein	22.80 a	22.88 a	23.90 b	0.80
ether extract	3.19 a	2.24 b	0.90 c	0.67
Water losses				
after cooking in water bath %	26.04 a	28.42 b	33.36 c	4.16
by pressure cm^2	9.94 a	10.37 a	11.76 b	1.89
WB force				
on raw meat kg	9.81 a	8.97	8.00 b	2.14
on cooked meat kg	10.59	10.67	10.42	2.15
Salting loss in ham %	1.97 a	2.47 b	2.61 b	0.60

Means with different letters differ at the 5% level.

Comparison between free-range and intensive system
Undoubtedly the future of the *Cinta Senese* breed is linked to extensive systems. These should allow the economic valorisation of marginal areas and the qualification of typical products. However, these production systems require longer productive cycles and proper feed management during certain periods of the year. Table 3 shows that CS-OUT reached slaughter weight 200 days later than CS-IN, with carcasses richer in fat cuts and poorer in lean cuts because of the high feeding input (availability of chestnuts and acorns) during the late fattening period. Differences between sexes were limited to higher dressing percentage and lower bone cuts in females.

Table 3. Slaughter traits of Cinta Senese pigs, in the two rearing systems: means and r. s. d.

	Rearing system		r.s.d.
	CS-IN	CS-OUT	
Age d	312 a	509 b	16.2
Slaughter weight kg	135.30 a	127.30 b	8.96
Dressing %	81.22	81.64	1.62
Lean cuts %	57.76 a	54.05 b	1.87
Fat cuts %	36.69 a	40.97 b	2.10
Bone cuts %	5.14	4.94	0.43

Means with different letters differ at the 5% level.

The effects of the rearing system on meat characteristics of *Cinta Senese* pigs are shown in table 4. No differences in pH were observed, while several authors found, on improved breeds, lower pH when the animals were raised outdoor (Van der Wal *et al.*, 1993; Sather *et al.*, 1997; Enfält *et al.*, 1997). However, it should be noted that in our study differences in feeding, season and age at slaughtering might have influenced this parameter. Meat of CS-OUT pigs was darker and more intensely coloured then that of CS-IN pigs, possibly due to older age and consequently higher myoglobin concentration (Mayoral *et al.,* 1999). Nevertheless it is known that animals of the same age reared under extensive versus intensive conditions have meat with higher chroma linked to increased exercise (Sather *et al.,* 1997). CS-OUT pigs had higher intramuscular fat, lower water holding capacity and firmer meat after cooking. Lower water holding capacity and firmer texture in outdoor versus indoors reared pigs have been also recorded in improved breeds (Sather *et al.,* 1997; Enfält *et al.,* 1997).

Table 4. Meat quality traits in Cinta Senese pigs in two rearing systems: means and r. s. d.

	Rearing system		r.s.d.
	CS-IN	CS-OUT	
pH$_{45}$	6.22	6.24	0.24
pH$_{24}$	5.78	5.83	0.18
Colour			
L*	49.70 a	46.46 b	3.64
chroma	12.38 a	15.57 b	2.05
hue	0.38	0.37	0.07
On wet basis %			
moisture	73.25 a	71.75 b	1.21
protein	22.78	23.02	1.00
ether extract	3.19 a	4.17 b	0.84
Water losses			
after cooking in water bath %	26.04 a	28.12 b	4.24
by pressure cm^2	9.94	9.55	1.73
WB force			
on raw meat kg	9.74	9.83	2.55
on cooked meat kg	10.53 a	15.02 b	2.75
Salting loss in ham %	2.01 a	4.29 b	0.89

Means with different letters differ at the 5% level.

2.2. Nera Siciliana breed

Experimental procedure
Forty castrated male and female *Nera Siciliana* pigs were reared with two different systems: (i) thirty one animals were reared following the traditional free-range farming, with little feed supplementation during summer; (ii) nine animals were reared in pens and were fed commercial mixture. Animals were slaughtered at 66 to 108 kg. of live body weight. Carcasses were dissected according to the "Modena" system and lean cuts (ham, shoulder, loin, neck), fat cuts (backfat, jowl, belly and kidney fat) and bone cuts (head and feet) were weighed. The *Longissimus lumborum* muscle (LL) was tested for: (i) pH$_{45}$ and pH$_{24}$; (ii) colour (CIE L*, a*, b*); (iii) chemical composition (A.O.A.C., 1980); (iv) water holding capacity determined as cooking loss percentage in oven and in water-bath (meat was cooked until the centre temperature reached 75°C); (v) shear force (Warner-Bratzler, Instron) on raw and cooked meat. Statistical analyses were carried out by GLM procedure (SAS, 1996).

Performance in the free-range system

In the traditional free-range farming, pigs are slaughtered at various ages and weights, depending on season (winter is preferred) and market offer. We investigated the joint effects of age and weight on carcass composition and meat quality. Curves were generated by quadratic equations in age and weight at slaughter. Figures 2 illustrate how carcass parameters are expected to vary as a function of age (from 420 to 480 days) and body weight (from 66 to 103 kg.). Dressing percentage increases with both body weight and age, but in younger animals where it decreases at higher body weights. Trends are similar for fat cuts percentage and are opposite for lean and bone cuts percentage. Then, in the *Nera Siciliana* breed reared under free-range conditions higher growth rate before fourteen months of age corresponds to proper lean and bone tissue growth and a consequent reduction of dressing percentage. When animals have to be slaughtered at an older age, as body weight increases fat deposition is more evident and killing out percentage increases.

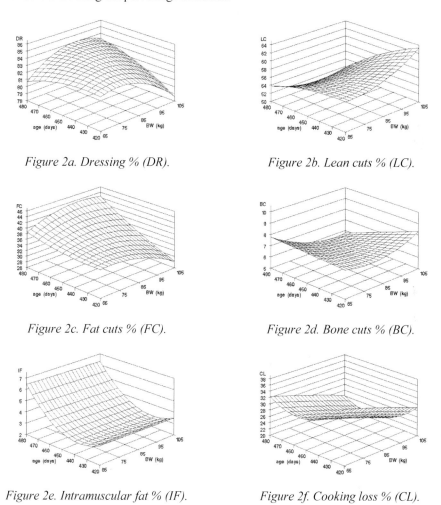

Figure 2a. Dressing % (DR).   Figure 2b. Lean cuts % (LC).

Figure 2c. Fat cuts % (FC).   Figure 2d. Bone cuts % (BC).

Figure 2e. Intramuscular fat % (IF).   Figure 2f. Cooking loss % (CL).

Figure 2. Trends of carcass and meat quality traits as a function of age (in days) and body weight (BW in kg) in Nera Siciliana.

The effects of age and body weight on two meat quality parameters are also illustrated in figures 2. Intra-muscular fat does not vary with body weight and increases somehow exponentially with age. Intra-muscular fat is 3% in younger animals and increases to 6% in pigs of 16 months of age. Cooking loss in oven, which is a measure of water holding capacity, decreases with increasing body weight and age; considering age, the decrease is mainly from 14 to 15 months.

Comparison between free-range and intensive system
Pigs reared in pens reached a body weight of 100 kg at almost thirteen months of age, approximately three months before the pigs reared in the traditional free-range system (table 5). These results show that the *Nera Siciliana*, compared to the *Cinta Senese*, is a late maturing pig of relative small size, with growth performance similar to those registered in the Corsican pig (Secondi *et al.*, 1996). Dressing percentage was higher in the free-ranging animals, possibly linked to their older age. No differences in carcass composition were observed between rearing systems.

Table 5. Slaughter traits of Nera Siciliana pigs in two rearing systems: means and r.s.d.

	Rearing system		r.s.d.
	indoor	outdoor	
Age d	380 a	452 b	22.40
Slaughter weight kg	96.2 a	86.3 b	8.10
Dressing %	81.10 a	82.85 b	1.75
Lean cuts %	55.90	55.10	3.66
Fat cuts %	37.35	38.14	4.12
Bone cuts %	6.75	6.77	0.75

Means with different letters differ at the 5% level.

Parameters of meat quality are shown in table 6. Values of pH_{45} are important because they assess the rate of fall of muscle pH and are good indicators of the pale, soft and exudative (PSE) meat condition. Both pH_{45} means were clearly above the critical threshold of 5.8, however a total of six animals showed quite low pH values. This may suggest to investigate for the possible presence in the population of the n mutation at the halothane sensitivity gene. Significant differences were registered between rearing systems for ultimate pH. Free-ranging pigs had a lower fall of pH, similarly to the observations in the *Cinta Senese* breed. Seven free-ranging pigs exceeded the threshold for ultimate pH of 6.2, indicative of meat classified as DFD. The use of DFD meat is not advisable in manufacturing cured hams, because it is linked to texture modifications and higher percentage of non edible hams (Guerrero *et al.*, 1999). Protein percentage was higher in indoor reared pigs, which showed lower contents of intramuscular fat, similarly to what observed in the *Cinta Senese*. Average intramuscular fat content of *Nera Siciliana* pigs was higher than that usually reported for breeds known for high intramuscular fat percentage, like *Duroc* and *Meishan*, although Lo *et al.* (1992) reported a *Duroc* line with almost 5% of intramuscular fat. High intramuscular fat was observed in several local breeds such as *Gascon* and *Limousin* (Simon *et al.*, 1996), Corsican (Coutron-Gambotti *et al.*, 1996) and Iberian (Serra *et al.*, 1998). With respect to meat colour, pigs reared in the outdoor system showed the lowest values of L and hue, in accordance with the results on the *Cinta Senese* breed. Outdoor rearing, possibly in relation to the older age at slaughter, resulted into darker and less yellow meat. In addition, this meat showed higher water holding capacity (after cooking in oven) and it had higher shear force value both before and after cooking.

Table 6. Meat quality traits in Nera Siciliana pigs in two rearing systems: means and r.s.d.

| | Rearing system | | r.s.d. |
	indoor	outdoor	
pH_{45}	6.07	6.15	0.29
pH_{24}	5.51 a	5.96 b	0.26
Colour			
L*	52.16 a	48.87 b	3.41
chroma	15.01	14.94	2.33
hue	0.39 a	0.34 b	0.07
On wet basis %			
moisture	72.18	72.44	1.21
protein	23.39 a	22.31 b	1.35
ether extract	3.15 a	4.58 b	0.68
Water losses			
after cooking in water bath %	26.70	26.40	5.78
after cooking in oven %	36.90 a	28.80 b	3.52
WB force			
on raw meat kg	6.15 a	10.62 b	3.21
on water bath cooked meat kg	8.12 a	12.26 b	2.43
on oven cooked meat kg	9.19 a	12.60 b	2.37

Means with different letters differ at the 5% level.

3. Reproduction traits

In tables 7 and 8 the reproductive performance of the five local breeds Calabrese, Casertana, *Cinta Senese*, *Nera Siciliana* and Mora Romagnola are shown. Reproduction traits are not routinely recorded in these breeds. The values reported in the tables are estimated on a limited number of litters because of the difficulty of monitoring reproduction in the free-range farming system (*Nera Siciliana*), the practice of crossbreeding which leads to few purebred litters (*Cinta Senese*) and the very small number of sows mated per year (Calabrese, Casertana, Mora Romagnola).

Table 7. Reproduction traits in Italian local pig breeds: means ± sd and range.

Breed	N.	Parity	Litter size	Born alive
Calabrese	7	all	3.9±1.1; 3-6	3.4±1.5; 1-6
Casertana	13	all	6.0±2.1; 4-10	4.4±2.9; 1-9
Cinta Senese	24	1st	6.6±1.8; 1-13	6.1±2.2; 1-13
	76	>1st	7.2±2.4; 1-14	7.1±2.5; 1-14
Nera Siciliana	14	1st	5.4±2.8; 1-11	5.2±2.9; 1-11
	26	>1st	8.3±2.4; 4-14	8.1±2.4; 4-14
Mora Romagnola	12	all	6.7±2.5; 2-10	6.1±3.1; 2-10

Mean litter size is 7 or lower in all breeds, but in the *Nera Siciliana*. Nevertheless in almost all breeds we observe litters with 10 or more piglets. In the *Nera Siciliana* there is a remarkable difference between first and higher parities (5.54±2.8 *vs.* 8.3±2.4), which is possibly related to the fact that females in the free-range system often mate at a very young age. In the Calabrese, Casertana and Mora Romagnola breeds performances should be interpreted with caution due to the small number of observations. In these breeds, considering the extremely small population sizes during the last years (see chapter 1.4), low performances could be related to inbreeding depression and absence of selection in the female renewal. In all breeds litter size might be also negatively affected by the relatively high age of breeding sows. Weaning percentage differs among breeds. The very low value (53%) observed in the Mora Romagnola might be both related to inbreeding depression and to poor management. Inbreeding might affect weaning success also in the *Cinta Senese*. In this breed we often observed a remarkable difference in morbidity and mortality between purebred piglets and crosses with Large White raised under same management conditions. In the *Nera Siciliana*, which is farmed under free-range conditions, as already discussed for litter size, there is a certain difference in the number of weaned piglets between first and higher parities. Finally, mean numbers of teats are 11,2±0.8, 10.1±1, 11±0.7 in *Nera Siciliana*, Casertana and Calabrese respectively. From 2000 the Pig Pedigree Registry requires that registered females in all five breeds have at least 10 teats.

Table 8. Reproduction traits in Italian local pig breeds: means ± sd and range.

Breed	N.	Parity	Birth weight (g)		Weaned piglets
Calabrese	7	all	1,195±186;	900-1,375	3.4±1.8; 1-6
Casertana	13	all	1,230±113;	1,025-1,460	4.2±3.1; 1-9
Cinta Senese	24	1st			4.0±2.8; 0-12
	76	>1st	1,330±301;	960-1,900	5.0±2.7; 0-12
Nera Siciliana	14	1st	1,170±460;	600-1,600	3.3±3.4; 0-11
	26	>1t	1,470±190;	970-1,650	6.2±2.6; 0-11
Mora Romagnola	12	all	1,260±220;	890-1530	3.2±3.3; 0-8

Finally it must be noted that in order to control inbreeding and genetic drift and to reduce the risk of extinction in the Calabrese, Casertana and Mora Romagnola breeds it is imperative to rapidly increase their population numbers. The low number of weaned piglets registered in these breeds during the last four years, possibly related to both inbreeding depression (*e.g.* Falconer, 1989) and poor management, might impair their capacity to recover from the present extremely low population sizes.

Acknowledgements

This work was financed by CE Regulation 1467/94, Contract RESGEN12.

Chapter 2.4. Performances of the Iberian and other local breeds of Spain

C. Barba[1], J.V. Delgado[1], J.R.B. Sereno[1], E. Dieguez[2], J. Forero[3], J. Jaume[4] and B. Peinado[5]

[1]*Unidad de Veterinaria. Departamento de Genética. Universidad de Córdoba (Spain)*
[2]*Breeder Association of Iberian Pig of Spain (AECERIBER)*
[3]*Área de Desarrollo Ganadero. Excma. Diputación Provincial de Huelva (Spain)*
[4]*Instituto de Biología Animal. Islas Baleares (Spain)*
[5]*Centro de Investigacion y Desarollo Agroalimentaria. Murcia (Spain)*

1. Introduction

The Iberian pig is responsible for more than ninety-nine per cent of the pig meat generated from native breeds in Spain. As explained in chapter 1.5 of this book, this production derives from several varieties, but at present most production comes from only a few of these varieties.

In this chapter we describe the productive performance of Iberian pig varieties and other Spanish native pig breeds. Most of the data presented here have been obtained by our team under the EU Project RESGEN12, but we present a review of this area in Spain, mentioning results of other authors. The presentation is divided into three sections: qualitative and quantitative body traits; growth and carcass traits and reproductive traits.

2. Qualitative and quantitative body traits

Anatomy and appearance were studied with a double purpose: the first being the relationship of these traits to production and product value, and the second the characterisation of Iberian varieties and other Spanish breeds based on morphological traits.

2.1. Iberian pig varieties and *Manchado de Jabugo*

In the Iberian pig studies we have worked with samples of unequal size, due to large differences in population size between varieties. This study covered two separate groups of characters. We used 7 qualitative (front profile, coat colour, hoof colour, etc) and 17 quantitative traits measured on 566 females belonging to 28 different herds, representing 7 Iberian varieties and the *Manchado de Jabugo* breed.

The statistical analysis was made in three steps: calculation of the descriptive statistics, comparison between populations for individual variables and multivariate analysis (canonical discriminant analysis and calculation of Mahalanobis distances). The differentiation among most of the varieties based on qualitative traits was clear. The study based on quantitative traits (Mata *et al.*, 1998; Pardo *et al.*, 1998 and Delgado *et al.*, 2000b) gave similar results. In Table 1, the means are presented, showing at a glance the clear differences observed in some of these variables. Table 2 shows the results of the Mahalanobis distances calculated using these traits (Delgado *et al.*, 1998). The multivariate analysis results showed a clear differentiation of *Manchado de Jabugo* for both qualitative and quantitative traits, as might be expected. The *Torbiscal* strain was clearly differentiated for qualitative traits only.

Table 1. Means and within-variety standard deviations (SD) for quantitative traits measured in adults (>2 years) of the Iberian pig varieties.

Variable (cm)	MA	EN	RP	MJ	RE	NI	SI	TO	SD
Numbers	103	240	59	16	155	91	21	96	--
Weight	119.8	122.8	104.9	101.8	137.0	144.9	118.5	131.2	28.41
Head width	13.3	13.7	13.0	13.3	13.6	13.8	13.2	13.9	1.36
Width between eyes	10.8	10.9	10.2	11.0	11.1	11.1	11.2	11.8	1.13
Ear width	11.3	11.5	11.2	12.0	11.5	12.7	12.0	12.8	1.39
Head length	32.0	31.6	29.3	27.1	30.7	31.1	30.0	31.3	2.99
Snout length	21.6	20.3	19.5	17.5	21.0	20.4	20.	22.0	2.11
Ear length	17.6	18.3	16.8	17.0	18.5	19.3	19.1	19.4	1.98
Height at withers	77.0	77.4	70.7	75.9	76.4	77.4	77.4	78.1	4.72
Height at beginning of rump	83.0	79.9	76.1	80.0	80.9	81.0	81.7	81.3	4.39
Rump width	20.0	22.1	17.4	27.6	23.2	24.4	22.1	22.1	3.09
Rump distance	13.5	13.8	11.9	14.4	14.3	15.2	14.2	14.9	1.68
Height of the rump	62.6	61.7	58.8	58.9	62.8	63.0	60.9	61.9	4.72
Rump at beginning of tail	30.6	29.3	29.5	30.7	31.2	32.5	29.1	32.1	3.69
Ham length	37.8	39.9	33.5	35.9	40.3	42.0	44.1	43.6	4.48
Shoulder length	20.3	20.1	22.0	24.2	20.7	20.8	20.8	21.1	2.86
Snack perimeter	15.3	15.5	15.2	16.6	15.8	15.7	15.7	16.3	0.89

Variety code: MA: Mamellado; EN: Entrepelado; RP: Retinto Portugués; MJ: Manchado de Jabugo; RE: Retinto; NI: Lampiño/Negro Iberico; SI: Silvela and TO: Torbiscal.

Table2. Mahalanobis distances among population using qualitative (above the diagonal) and quantitative traits (below the diagonal).

	MA	EN	RP	MJ	RE	NI	SI	TO
MA		3.899***	6.914***	56.090***	1.941^{ns}	9.906***	4.887**	68.933***
EN	2.502^{ns}		1.813**	57.669***	3.859***	4.489***	7.301***	69.921***
RP	6.240*	9.853***		59.168***	3.285***	0.649^{ns}	4.812***	65.372***
MJ	29.543***	23.39***	26.83***		52.613***	58.780***	54.028***	30.869***
RE	3.0669^{ns}	1.282***	10.93***	23.45***		4.121***	1.199^{ns}	61.108***
NI	6.966***	3.325***	15.81***	25.27***	2.198***		4.600***	62.936***
SI	6.178*	2.659**	15.58***	24.63***	3.154***	4.636***		51.929***
TO	5.057**	3.262***	14.48***	26.99***	2.67***	3.708***	1.622^{ns}	

Variety code: see Table 1.
Levels of significance: ns not significant, *P< 0.05, **P<0.01, and ***P<0.001.

In the variance analysis among varieties for individual variables, we observed that significant differences were evident in most of the traits studied. The homogeneity group established with the Duncan test (Delgado at al., 2000b) demonstrated that *Manchado de Jabugo* was clearly differentiated, and varieties such as *Torbiscal, Entrepelado* and *Lampiño* were responsible for a large part of the variance. The population structure of the Iberian pig determined by clustering methods based on quantitative variation confirmed the differentiation of *Manchado de Jabugo*.

2.2. Negro Canario

In the *Negro Canario* pig Lopez *et al.* (1992) developed the first deep zoometric work in the Spanish pig breeds. Their results are shown in table 3.

Table 3. Means and within-sex standard deviations (SD) observed in the quantitative study of adult animals (> 2 years) of Negro Canario.

Variable (cm)	Males	Females	SD
Numbers	4	7	--
Height at withers	87.2	81.1	11.41
Height at back	86.2	83.9	9.31
Height at head of tail	72.5	66.3	10.97
Oblique length	104.5	99.7	8.88
Straight thoracic perimeter	142.2	131.9	9.89
Oblique thoracic perimeter	155	138.9	10.41
Depth of chest	47.7	48.1	4.23
Occipital coccyx length	145.5	132.8	6.60
Width between eyes	9.7	9.7	14.78
Length of head	30.2	27.7	6.21
Width of head	13	10.7	10.62
Length of rump	30.4	30.3	12.69
Width across hips	26.5	26.3	11.20
Perimeter of metacarpian	24.7	22.7	11.76
Width across 6th rib	35	31.9	7.45
Length of ham	47.5	44.1	10.51

2.3. Chato Murciano

Some data from a small sample of the *Chato Murciano* breed (12 females) have also been published by our team (Poto *et al.,* 2000). We studied head length (25.65 cm), head width (16.32 cm), length of snout (8.5 cm), distance between eyes (11.91 cm), height at withers (65.25 cm), rump width (33.12 cm), longitudinal diameter (97.75 cm), Breast height (37.87 cm), Breast width (31.93 cm), height to rump (71.12 cm), rump length (28.33 cm), thoracic circumference (112.87 cm) and shank circumference (18 cm). Also the number of teats was registered with values between 12 and 14 and around a mean of 12.7.

3. Growth and carcass traits

3.1. Iberian pig varieties

The productive characterisation of 6 Iberian pig varieties (Barba, 1999) was based on the performances of individual pigs during three periods of their productive life: from birth to start of fattening (2059 animals from 18 herds), from start to end of fattening (1359 animals from 28 herds) and at slaughter (1359 animals from 28 herds) We studied weights at different ages between birth and slaughter and daily gains between different ages.

In table 4 we present the mean values of the different traits observed in each of the three periods studied. From this table we can expect some productive specialisation of the Iberian varieties studied. Table 5 shows the Mahalanobis distances obtained in the multivariate analysis developed in each of the three periods. In general we can say that the Iberian pig varieties present clear productive specialisation. In the pre-weaning period the *Retinto* and *Portugues* varieties were seen to be best in terms of growth capacity, so they were considered the most developed varieties.

Table 4. *Means and within-variety standard deviations (SD) of growth and carcass traits in the Iberian pig varieties.*

	Test				Variety				SD
Variable		MA	EN	RP	RE	NI	SI	TO	
First period									
Numbers		201	441	210	538	231	438	--	--
Birth weight (kg)	**	1.24	1.40	1.14	1.50	1.32	1.28	--	0.27
Weight (kg)at 60 days	**	13.91	11.56	15.58	14.63	13.77	13.13	--	4.68
Daily gain (g) 0-60 days	**	231.00	192.50	429.30	246.10	229.30	218.40	--	79.61
Second period									
Numbers		39	136	--	352	32	158	131	--
Weight (kg) at 150 days	***	46.26	49.39	--	47.92	58.47	48.43	55.72	11.09
Weight (kg) at 360 days	***	111.00	118.50	--	115.00	140.30	116.20	133.70	26.62
Weight (kg) at 450 days	***	159.20	170.70	--	166.70	183.50	167.90	191.20	26.57
Daily gain (g) 150-360 days	***	308.40	392.30	--	319.40	389.80	322.80	371.50	86.23
Daily gain (g) 360-450 days	***	581.40	579.00	--	579.10	487.80	576.40	636.70	146.50
Daily gain (g) 150-450 days	***	403.90	417.10	--	409.80	424.80	406.80	466.20	66.65
Third period									
Numbers		39	136	--	352	32	158	131	--
Carcass weight (kg)	***	134.10	143.20	--	139.40	159.40	136.40	157.50	22.48
Carcass yield relative to liveweight	***	0.83	0.84	--	0.84	0.87	0.81	0.83	3.46
Ham weight (kg)	***	20.50	21.28	--	21.10	22.42	21.31	24.99	3.43
Ham yield relative to carcass weight	***	0.15	0.15	--	0.15	0.14	0.16	0.16	0.01
Shoulder blade weight (kg)	***	13.88	14.25	--	14.07	13.57	14.17	16.29	2.35
Shoulder blade yield relative to carcass weight	***	0.10	0.10	--	0.10	0.09	0.10	0.10	0.01
Noble pieces yield relative to carcass weight	***	0.25	0.25	--	0.25	0.23	0.26	0.26	0.02

Variety code: see Table 1.
Levels of significance: ** $P<0.01$ and *** $P<0.001$.

In the post-weaning period, the best varieties were *Lampiño* (*Negro Iberico*) and *Torbiscal*, the first in the pre-fattening period because the rusticity of this ancestral variety is very well adapted to the paddocks, the second in the fattening period because it is the most selected variety. The latter period corresponds to the introduction of the animals in the extensive systems, some varieties showing better adaptation than others to the primary assimilation of acorn feeding. The slaughter variables showed important differences regarding carcass quality, taking into account their yields in noble pieces. *Lampiño* (*Negro Iberico*) gave the best carcass yield, but *Torbiscal* and *Silvela* offered the highest yield of noble pieces.

Table 5. Mahalanobis distances among Iberian pig varieties using pre-weaning (line 1), post-weaning (line 2) (above the diagonal) and slaughter traits (line 1 below the diagonal).

		SI	RE	TO	NI	EN	MA	RP
SI	1		1.30***	-	0.15*	0.03 ns	0.45***	10.20***
	2		1.01***	2.12**	2.71***	1.07***	0.50 ns	-
RE	1	0.14*		-	0.79***	1.62***	1.19***	8.61***
	2			1.06***	1.20***	0.02 ns	2.68***	-
TO	1	1.64***	1.71***		-	-	-	-
	2				1.19***	0.77***	4.64***	-
NI	1	3.46***	2.58***	3.15***		0.29***	0.14*	8.13***
	2					0.99***	4.90***	-
EN	1	0.79***	0.34***	2.08***	2.24***		0.65***	11.10***
	2						2.88***	-
MA	1	0.16 ns	0.14 ns	2.37***	3.67***	0.48 ns		6.38***
	2							
RP		-	-	-	-	-	-	-

Variety code: see Table 1.
Levels of significance: ns not significant, * P<0.05, ** P<0.01 and *** P<0.001.

3.2. Manchado de Jabugo

We have considered the growth performances of *Manchado de Jabugo* (Forero, 1999 and Forero *et al.*, 1999) in a separate study on 140 animals from two herds. In table 6 we show the descriptive statistics for birth weight, weight at 60 days and daily gain 0-60 days by sex. Additionally, an analysis of variance of these variables including the fixed effects of sex, year and parity number showed significant effects of parity for all variables, and significant effects of sex in birth weight only, and of year in daily gain only.

Table 6. Growth performances of Manchado de Jabugo males and females (means ± standard error).

Variable	Males	Females
Numbers	73	67
Birth weight (kg)	1.66±0.03	1.54±0.03
Weight at 60 days (kg)	12.50±0.44	12.52±0.42
Daily gain 0-60 d (g)	202.9±5.88	209.53±6.04

3.3. Chato Murciano

Peinado *et al.* (1999) have studied the growth performance of the *Chato Murciano* breed, using a sample of 242 pure animals of the breed. Birth weight was around 1.41 kg, but depended on litter size (1.57 - 0.96 kg). The weight at the beginning of the dry feeding was 2.87 kg and the weaning weight (21-26 days) was around 6.6 kg. These authors also registered the performances during fattening. The daily gain throughout the fattening period was 478 g./day, with an evident sexual dimorphism (323 g for females and 518 g for males). The feed conversion index was also studied, giving values of 2.68 and 3.3 kg of food per kg of body weight in males and females respectively.

3.4. Negre Mallorqui

The growth performance of the *Negre Mallorqui* breed was studied by Jaume *et al.* (1999) but under special feeding conditions, using dry meal of carob beans. The authors monitored the growth of 68 piglets from eight different litters between birth and weaning. The weaning weight observed was 7.4 kg, showing a daily gain of 162 g and a food conversion index of 1.34 kg food/kg of body weight. Birth weight was not mentioned.

3.5. Negro Canario

For the *Negro Canario* breed, the DAD-IS database (see Appendix of chapter 1.1) mentions some performance values: 1.2 kg and 1.35 kg, for birth weight of males and females respectively. 250 g for daily gain during the fattening period, and 40 % of lean meat in the carcass.[Consultation of 3 Nov 2000].

4. Reproductive traits

4.1. Iberian pig varieties and Manchado de Jabugo

We have studied the reproductive traits of Iberian pig females belonging to several varieties (Suarez *et al.*, 2000). In this study we measured total piglets born, piglets born alive and piglets weaned in 532 litters. Table 7 shows descriptive statistics of these three variables in each populations. Generally there existed differences in reproductive performances. *Torbiscal* and *Manchado de Jabugo* were observed to feature about 1.5 piglets above the mean for number born alive, while at weaning the differences were reduced to 0.75 and 0.4 in the two afore-mentioned populations respectively. These populations showed a higher prolificacy, but their maternal abilities were not as good. *Negro Iberico* is one of the most primitive variety, and showed the worst reproductive performances.

Table 7. Descriptive statistics of reproductive traits in the Iberian pig varieties.

Variety	piglets born		piglets born alive		piglets weaned	
	N	Mean±S.Error	N	Mean±S.Error	N	Mean±S.Error
Torbiscal	17	8.35±0.45	17	7.82±0.45	17	6.82±0.33
Lampino/Negro Iberico	17	5.53±0.32	11	5.82±0.40	17	4.94±0.44
Mamellado	54	6.09±0.22	50	6.00±0.22	54	6.02±0.22
Silvela	186	6.38±0.15	158	6.11±0.13	186	6.03±0.14
Retinto	140	6.31±0.16	135	6.29±0.16	140	6.24±0.16
Entrepelado	50	6.04±0.16	43	6.07±0.18	50	5.84±0.18
Portugués	20	6.00±0.29	20	6.00±0.29	20	6.00±0.29
M. Jabugo	48	8.10±0.29	48	7.81±0.25	48	6.46±0.25
Total	532	6.45±0.08	482	6.34±0.08	532	6.07±0.08

4.2. Chato Murciano

Peinado *et al.* (1999) also studied reproductive performances in the *Chato Murciano* breed. They found a mean litter size of 7.66 piglets born, with a mean value of 6.68 for piglets born alive and a value of 4.61 piglets weaned. In this breed we observed an acceptable prolificacy but the high level of inbreeding might have impaired weaning performances, with a loss of around two piglets per litter under the mother's care.

4.3. Negre Mallorqui

In *Negre Mallorqui*, Jaume *et al.* (1999) observed 273 litters of 32 sows, with a mean value of 2.13 litters per sow per year. The registered prolificacy was 7.74 piglets at birth, 7.43 born alive, and 6.03 weaned. In this paper the authors studied several fixed, random and co-variable effects over these variables.

5. Conclusions

Our results on the morphological, productive and reproductive characterisation of the Iberian pig varieties have demonstrated the existence of large differences among populations within the Iberian pig branch. These differences highlight the interesting genetic diversity of the Iberian pig which allows exploitation in extensive conditions in diverse environments, as well as offering the market a diversity of products. The differentiation of *Manchado de Jabugo* was also clearly determined as a separate breed. Some authors in Spain have considered this breed as another variety of the Iberian pig. Our results rejected this hypothesis absolutely.

These results have been presented to official Spanish institutions in order to get support for the correct genetic management of the Spanish native breeds. The productive characterisation of these populations is important for demonstrating their specific adaptations. Their conservation can thus be justified and their competitive introduction into the free market may be assisted by official financial compensations and supported by protected product trade mark

SECTION III

EVALUATION OF GENETIC DIVERSITY AMONG EUROPEAN BREEDS (GENETIC DISTANCES)

Chapter 3.1. Evaluation of genetic diversity from immunological, biochemical and DNA polymorphisms

L. Ollivier[1], J.-C. Caritez[2], J.-L. Foulley[1], C. Legault[1], M. San Cristobal-Gaudy[3], F. Labroue[4], Y. Amigues[5], H. Brandt[6], R. Clemens[6], P. Glodek[6], P. Ludewig[6], C. Kaltwasser[6], J.-N. Meyer[6], R. Davoli[7], G. Gandini[8], A. Martinez[9], J.L. Vega-Pla[10] and J.V. Delgado[9]

[1]*INRA- Station de Génétique Quantitative et Appliquée, 78350 Jouy-en-Josas, France*
[2]*INRA- Domaine pluridisciplinaire du Magneraud, 17700 Surgères, France*
[3]*INRA- Laboratoire de Génétique Cellulaire, BP 26, 31326 Castanet-Tolosan cedex, France*
[4]*Institut Technique du Porc, BP 3, 35651 Le Rheu cedex, France*
[5]*Labogena, 78350 Jouy-en-Josas*
[6]*Institute of Animal Breeding and Genetics, University of Göttingen, Albrecht-Thaer Weg 3, 37075 Göttingen, Germany*
[7]*DIPROVAL, Università di Bologna, Via Rosselli 107, 42100 Reggio Emilia, Italy*
[8]*Istituto de Zootecnica, Università di Milano, Via Celoria 10, 20133 Milano, Italy*
[9]*Departamento de Genetica, Universidad de Cordoba, Avenida Medina Azahara, 14004 Cordoba, Spain*
[10]*Laboratorio de Grupos Sanguineos. Cria Caballar, Apartado Oficial Sucursal 2, 14071 Cordoba, Spain*

1. Introduction

The efficient management and use of genetic resources imply their being characterised as comprehensively as possible. Characterisation may be performed in various ways. First, breed inventories and collection of minimum population data (also called "passport data") can give an overview of the whole range of resources available in a given species. This aspect was addressed in the first section of this book on *primary characterisation*. Whenever possible, primary characterisation has to be completed by more detailed information on breed similarities, in terms of *reproductive and productive performances*, as done in the second section. In this third section characterisation at genome level will be attempted. Genetic markers have been used for nearly 40 years in farm animal species for studying between breed variation. They have the advantage of allowing a direct evaluation of *genetic diversity*, by definition free of any environmental effect. The purpose of this section is to present results on various genetic polymorphisms in the breeds of the RESGEN project, and to evaluate their genetic diversity based on the genetic distances among them.

2. Review of the literature on comparisons among European breeds of pigs

For a long time research on genetic polymorphisms in farm animals has been limited to erythrocyte antigens or *blood groups*. A major breakthrough appeared with starch gel electrophoresis and a wealth of polymorphic protein systems, so called *biochemical polymorphisms*, were then evidenced. A historical overview and a presentation of the pig immunological and biochemical polymorphisms in the early 1980s has been published by Ollivier and Sellier (1983). In the meantime, considerable efforts were devoted to gene mapping. However, gene maps remained rudimentary until the early 1990s and the genome position of the loci studied was mostly unknown. Since then, the identification of genes and genetic markers based on *DNA sequence* variation has resulted in a rapid increase in genome coverage in the pig, like in most other species of farm animals. Detailed porcine linkage maps mainly including microsatellites have been published (Archibald *et al.*, 1995 ; Rohrer *et al.*, 1996). Such maps have also allowed several blood group and biochemical polymorphism loci to be now accurately mapped (Rohrer *et al.*, 1997).

Attempts to utilise genetic markers for comparing breeds of pigs started in the 1960s. The first studies were those of Major (1968) on the use of blood groups for comparing various European *Landraces*, and of Dinklage and Gruhn (1969) on blood groups and serum proteins applied to German breeds. An extensive literature has also been devoted over the last 30 years to comparing wild boars and domesticated breeds from various continents, with a view to tracing the possible origin of our present breeds. These aspects will not be covered in this review, since our emphasis is primarily on the evaluation of genetic diversity within the European continent.

Table 1 summarises some comparisons of European breeds published over the last decade. The table shows a variety of approaches, implying highly variable numbers of individuals sampled per breed (n), of marker loci (L) and of alleles per locus (k). In a report to FAO, Barker *et al.* (1993) proposed an expression for the coefficient of variation of the estimated distance, intended for designing such programmes, which is applied in table 1. A detailed derivation of this formula, and its implications have recently been provided by Foulley and Hill (1999). The report of Barker *et al.* (1993) also emphasised the need to co-ordinate microsatellite typing across different laboratories and particularly to ensure that the same microsatellite loci and alleles are typed in all laboratories. Consequently, a panel of microsatellite markers was chosen for the pig following those recommendations, and further approved by the FAO-ISAG Advisory Committee for genetic distance studies. This panel was used in the PiGMaP pilot study carried over 1994-1996 (see Laval *et al.*, 2000) and in the study of Martinez *et al.* (2000b).

Table 1. Some studies of genetic distances (d) among European breeds of pigs.

Origin of breeds	Number of breeds	n average	n range	Polymorphisms	L	k	Coefficient of variation of d[1]	Reference
Belgium, Bulgaria and France	4	576	159-1227	BB	29	3.5	0.17	Van Zeveren et al. (1990)
Germany	14	226	100-404	BB	22	3.2	0.22	Glodek et al. (1993)
Belgium	4	187	122-213	MS	7	13.3	0.17	Van Zeveren et al. (1995)
Spain, Portugal (Iberian varieties), and Duroc	10	23	7-41	MS	25	8.2	0.20	Martinez et al. (2000b)
6 European countries and wild pig	11	44	9-56	MS	18	10.8	0.15	Laval et al. (2000)

[1] $(1 + 1/nd)[2/L(k-1)]^{0.5}$ (Barker et al., 1993; Foulley and Hill, 1999), assuming d (Sanghvi) = 0.05.

n: number of individuals sampled per breed;
L: number of marker loci;
k: average number of alleles per locus;
BB: blood groups and biochemical polymorphisms;
MS: microsatellites (simple DNA sequence repeat).

3. Genetic markers selected and typing techniques

The list of the genetic markers used in this project is given in table 2, which also indicates their assignment to the pig genome maps presently available. The techniques applied are briefly described below.

Table 2. Chromosome location of the marker loci used in the RESGEN[1] and PIGBIODIV[2] projects (based on Rohrer et al., 1996 and Rohrer et al., 1997).

Chromosome	Marker	Chromosome	Marker
1	**S0155**	8	PGM
	EAA		**S0225**
2	**SW240**		EAF*
	S0226		**S0178**
3	**S0002**	9	EAK
4	**S0227**		**SW911**
	EAL		EAE
5	**S0005**	10	**SW951**
	IGF1	12	EAD
6	EAS		**S0090**
	EAH	13	TF
	GPI		**S0215**
	PGD	14	**SW857**
	SW122	15	EAG
	EAO	17	**SW24**
7	**SW632**		EAI
	PI1		AMY
	PI2	X	**S0218**

In bold: 18 microsatellites belonging to the FAO-ISAG recommended panel.
Codes for markers: Blood groups (Erythrocyte Antigens): EAA, EAB, EAC, EAD, EAE, EAF, EAG, EAH, EAI, EAK, EAL, EAO, EAS. Biochemical polymorphisms (enzymes and serum proteins): ADA (Adenosine deaminase), AMY (Serum amylase), ESD (Esterase D), GPI (Glucose phosphate isomerase), PGI (Phosphogluconate dehydrogenase, PGM (Phosphoglucomutase), PI1, PI2, PI3 (Protease inhibitors), PO2A (Postalbumin 2A), TF (Transferrin). Microsatellites: S0155, SW240,... IGF1, etc...
*Provisional location.
Assigned: EAC to chromosome 7, ESD to chromosome 13.
Unassigned: ADA, EAB, PI3, PO2A.
[1]European Commission contract RESGEN-CT95-012.
[2]European Commission contract BIO4-CT98-0188.

3.1. Blood groups and biochemical polymorphisms

Blood samples of 3 German pig breeds (SH, BB and AS), 1 Czech (PR) and 1 Polish (PU) breed were collected in tubes with sodium-cyanide stabilisator and cooled at 4°C, until use in the laboratory of Göttingen. The samples were separated and aliquoted in plasma for serum proteins, erythrocytes for enzymes and 6% erythrocyte suspension for blood group typing. Plasma and erythrocyte samples of 2 Italian breeds (NS and MR) and 3 Spanish breeds (MJ, NI and RE) were also available.

Thirteen blood group systems (EAA/EAS, EAB, EAC, EAD, EAE, EAF, EAG, EAH, EAI, EAK, EAL and EAO) were tested on 5 breeds (German, Czech and Polish) following the ISAG comparison tests. Six serum protein systems (TF = Transferrin, AMY = Serum amylase, PI1/2/3 = Protease inhibitor1/2/3) and PO2A = Postalbumin 2A) could be analysed in all 10 breeds, while five enzyme systems (Adenosine deaminase = ADA, Esterase D = ESD, Glucosephosphate isomerase = GPI, Phosphogluconate dehydrogenase = PGD and Phosphoglucomutase = PGM) - except PGM, which could not be analysed in the Italian and Spanish breeds - were analysed (as described by Clemens and Meyer, 1996) in 9 breeds only, since no erythrocytes were available in NI. The number of samples and systems tested are shown in table 3, which shows the variation in tests available and sample size among the 10 breeds.

3.2. Microsatellites

From the initial panel of microsatellites mentioned above in 2, a subset of 18 markers was analysed in the study of Laval *et al.* (2000). The results from this study, on 5 of the breeds included in the RESGEN12 project, were combined with those of the Labogena laboratory of Jouy-en-Josas on the remaining 13 breeds (as a part of the pig genetic diversity study hereafter called PIGBIODIV). The 18 breeds covered are listed in table 3. Blood samples from the 13 PIGBIODIV breeds were collected by the participants from France (INRA), Germany (Göttingen), Italy (Bologna and Milano) and Spain (Cordoba), and DNA was extracted in the corresponding laboratories of INRA-Le Magneraud, Animal Genetics Institute of Göttingen, University of Bologna and Veterinary Faculty of Cordoba. The samples were all shipped to Labogena where they were analysed using an ABI 3700 fluorescent DNA sequencer (multi-capillary). Batches of 92 samples were genotyped together and completed with the 4 control animals from the PiGMaP reference families used previously by Laval *et al.* (2000). These control DNAs allowed to establish the correspondence between allele sizes at Labogena and in the study of Laval *et al.* (2000).

Table 3 summarises the markers used in this project, namely 13 blood groups, 11 biochemical polymorphisms and 18 microsatellites. The average within–breed genetic polymorphism is analysed in table 4. Though the 3 categories of genetic markers were not investigated on the same sample of breeds, the general tendency confirms the lower variability usually shown by blood groups and biochemical polymorphisms compared to microsatellites. For the latter, average allelic richness ranges from 3.1 in *Manchado de Jabugo* to 7.0 alleles per locus in *Créole* and average heterozygosity also shows large variation between breeds. It should be noted that the average number of microsatellite alleles per locus is more than doubled over the 18 breeds compared to the average within breed figure. An important between-breed component of allelic richness is thus exhibited in this category of markers, which appears to be relatively smaller in the 2 other categories.

Table 3. Number of individuals sampled for genetic distancing in the RESGEN and PIGBIODIV projects.

Country	Breed name[1]	Country-breed Code	Blood groups[2] (13 systems)	Biochemical polymorphisms[2] (11 systems)	Microsatellites (18 loci)	
					M	F
France	**Basque**	FRBA			22	25
	Blanc de l'Ouest	FRBO			21	31
	Créole	FRCR			14	25
	Gascon	FRGA			25	31
	Limousin	FRLI			27	29
Germany and Central Europe	Angler Sattelschwein	DEAS	60-71	56-71	17	39
	Bunte Bentheimer	DEBB	35-48	35-48	28	19
	Schwäbisch-Hällisches Schwein	DESH	144-145[3]	143-145[4]	29	25
	Presticke	CZPR	72-75	75	13	37
	Pulawska Spot	PLPU	78	68-78	24	24
Italy	Calabrese	ITCA	-	-	4	15
	Casertana	ITCT	-	-	12	16
	Cinta Senese	ITCS	-	-	15	15
	Mora Romagnola	ITMR	-	13-14[5]	-	-
	Nera Siciliana	ITNS	-	18-21[5]	26	24
Spain	Manchado de Jabugo	ESMJ	-	13-20[5]	18	18
	Negro Canario	ESNC	-	-	6	12
	Negro Iberico	ESNI	-	29-31[6]	45	3
	Retinto	ESRE	-	61-93[5]	43	25
Average sample size			83.4	59.6	21.6	22.9

M: males; F: females.
[1]In bold: breeds included in the PiGMaP pilot study of Laval et al. (2000).
[2]listed in table 2.
[3]12 for EAO.
[4]12 for PI3 and ESD.
[5]PGM excluded.
[6]ADA, ESD, GPI, PGD, and PGM excluded.

Table 4. Average number of alleles (n) and heterozygosity (H) observed (number of loci in brackets).

Breed[1]	Blood groups (13)		Biochemical polymorphisms (11)		Microsatellites (18)	
	n	H	n	H	n	H^2
FRBA	-	-	-	-	3.17	0.34
FRBO	-	-	-	-	4.17	0.52
FRCR	-	-	-	-	7.00	0.59
FRGA	-	-	-	-	4.06	0.46
FRLI	-	-	-	-	3.61	0.41
DEAS	2.69	0.43	2.18	0.31	5.56	0.63
DEBB	2.23	0.28	1.91	0.30	4.50	0.58
DESH	2.85	0.41	2.45	0.31	5.67	0.52
CZPR	2.85	0.34	2.00	0.30	5.94	0.63
PLPU	2.15	0.25	2.09	0.32	4.61	0.58
ITCA	-	-	-	-	2.78	0.47
ITCT	-	-	-	-	4.33	0.55
ITCS	-	-	-	-	4.17	0.47
ITMR	-	-	1.30	0.08	-	-
ITNS	-	-	2.20	0.20	6.72	0.59
ESMJ	-	-	1.70	0.22	3.11	0.42
ESNC	-	-	-	-	3.61	0.46
ESNI	-	-	2.00	0.20	4.94	0.54
ESRE	-	-	2.00	0.19	5.94	0.53
Within breed (overall) average	2.55 (3.00)	0.34	1.98 (2.73)	0.25	4.66 (10.20)	0.52

[1]breed codes as in table 3;
[2]females only for the X-linked marker S0218.

4. Genetic distances and genetic diversity

Genetic distances between breeds were calculated using the allelic frequencies for the markers shared in each breed combination. The same measures of distance as in Laval *et al.* (2000) were used, namely the distance of Reynolds *et al.* (1983) and the Nei standard distance (Nei, 1972). Two additional measures, the distance of Gregorius (1974) and Nei minimum (Nei, 1987), were applied to the blood groups and biochemical polymorphisms.

Table 5 presents the genetic distances (Reynolds and Nei standard) among the 19 breeds, separately for the blood group and biochemical polymorphisms (BB) on one line, and for the microsatellites (MS) on the other. Comparing the figures in the 2 lines clearly shows that the values of the Reynolds distances were of the same order for both types of markers (maximum 0.43 and 0.44). This confirms the expectation for this measure of distance not to be affected by the number of alleles (Laval *et al.*, 2001; Foulley unpublished results). In contrast, the Nei standard distances were markedly lower for BB (maximum 0.19) compared to MS (maximum 0.79). This distance is indeed dependent on the average level of heterozygosity (H), since its approximate expectation, as a function of H and F (Reynolds distance), can be shown to be $\log_e [1 + 2F H/(1-H)]^{0.5}$ (Laval *et al.*, 2001). Based on MS, the 2 largest distances involved the *Basque* (both for Reynolds and Nei). The 2 smallest Reynolds and Nei distances involved the same breed-combinations, the most closely related breeds being the red (*Retinto*) and black (*Negro Iberico*) Iberians followed by *Nera Siciliana* and *Créole*. Based on BB, the 2 largest distances, Reynolds as well as Nei, involved the *Mora Romagnola* (a breed not typed for MS), and the closest breeds were *Nera Siciliana* and *Retinto*, followed by *Angler Sattelschwein* and *Nera Siciliana*. Considering only the set of 8 breeds typed for both sets of markers, it appeared that the *Manchado de Jabugo* consistently showed the highest average distance to the other breeds whatever the type of marker.

Those genetic distances were used to measure diversity along the procedure suggested by Weitzman (1993). In our situation the method was applied to the evaluation of various patterns of potential breed extinction, as advocated by Thaon d'Arnoldi *et al.* (1998), by evaluating the contribution of each breed, or of each set of breeds belonging to a particular country, to the total diversity, as shown in table 6. This table clearly shows the unequal contributions of the various breeds to the total diversity. Based on the BB polymorphisms, the breeds marginal contributions ranged from approximately 1 % (ITNS) to 30 % (ITMR) of the 10 breeds diversity. Based on the MS polymorphisms, on a larger set of breeds, the range went from about 1 % (ESRE) to nearly 12 % (FRBA) of the 18 breeds diversity, bearing in mind the absence of the breed ITMR in the latter set. When the 2 measures of distances were compared, the ranking of the breeds appeared to be rather consistent for BB, which was not quite the case however for MS, where DESH appeared to contribute most to diversity based on Nei as against FRBA when Reynolds was considered. As to countries, the set of Italian and Spanish breeds chosen here appeared to contribute about equally to total diversity whether based on BB or on MS. Somewhat higher contributions from the German and Central European set for BB and from the French set for MS were also to be noted. It is worth mentioning that the country overall contributions may markedly differ from the sum of their breed contributions.

Table 5. Genetic distances between the 19 breeds[1] (18 microsatellite markers and 24 blood group and biochemical polymorphism systems[2]).

Breed	FRBA	FRBO	FRCR	FRGA	FRLI	DEAS	DEBB	DESH	CZPR	PLPU	ITCA	ITCT	ITCS	ITMR	ITNS	ESMJ	ESNC	ESNI	ESRE
FRBA	--	0.3397	0.2692	0.2725	0.4358	0.3118	0.3307	0.3589	0.2766	0.3019	0.4270	0.3176	**0.4396**	-	0.2761	**0.4406**	0.3938	0.3147	0.3160
FRBO	0.4536	--	0.1681	0.2714	0.3126	0.1929	0.2036	0.2552	0.1954	0.2382	0.2923	0.2918	0.2942	-	0.1706	0.3379	0.3179	0.2201	0.2125
FRCR	0.4196	0.2891	--	0.1485	0.1884	0.0898	0.1265	0.1457	0.0758	0.1089	0.1813	0.1443	0.1557	-	*0.0435*	0.1568	0.2029	0.1168	0.0889
FRGA	0.3205	0.4498	0.2583	--	0.2963	0.1687	0.2244	0.2382	0.1464	0.1905	0.2982	0.2516	0.2988	-	0.1647	0.3080	0.2642	0.2520	0.2309
FRLI	0.6696	0.4698	0.2835	0.4489	--	0.2057	0.2589	0.2886	0.1913	0.2386	0.3307	0.3359	0.2962	-	0.1964	0.3315	0.3483	0.2817	0.2717
DEAS	0.5253	0.3356	0.1895	0.2929	0.3097	--	0.1131	0.1688	0.0515	0.1097	0.2017	0.2209	0.2197	-	0.0861	0.2239	0.2416	0.1478	0.1430
DEBB	0.5072	0.3172	0.2402	0.3894	0.3951	0.1955	--	0.2082	0.1303	0.1444	0.2384	0.2405	0.2600	*0.3661*	0.1420	0.3024	0.2756	0.1991	0.1854
DESH	**0.7943**	0.5817	0.3922	0.5490	0.6113	0.4422	0.5035	--	0.1508	0.2022	0.2500	0.2286	0.2244	**0.4224**	0.1406	0.2775	0.2992	0.2064	0.1882
CZPR	0.4304	0.3551	0.1628	0.2476	0.2846	0.0965	0.2436	0.3956	--	0.0951	0.1943	0.1910	0.2047	*0.4102*	0.0821	0.1943	0.2244	0.1559	0.1575
PLPU	0.4342	0.4144	0.2034	0.3108	0.3526	0.1935	0.2383	0.4948	0.1674	--	0.2550	0.1219	0.2446	*0.3720*	0.1345	0.2273	0.2771	0.1913	0.1403
ITCA	0.6324	0.4135	0.2644	0.4513	0.4463	0.2980	0.3428	0.4582	0.2894	0.3911	--	0.2707	0.2434	-	0.1783	0.3281	0.2799	0.2452	0.2106
ITCT	0.5012	0.6269	0.3145	0.5064	0.7018	0.5563	0.5345	0.6523	0.4604	0.4796	0.4534	--	0.2618	-	0.1498	0.3268	0.2656	0.1767	0.1666
ITCS	**0.7814**	0.4721	0.2450	0.5133	0.4102	0.3939	0.4497	0.4388	0.3647	0.4149	0.2953	0.4884	--	-	0.1720	0.3081	0.3444	0.2074	0.1756
ITMR	-	-	-	-	-	-	-	-	-	-	-	-	-	--	0.3102	0.2543	-	0.0922	*0.0185*
ITNS	0.4325	0.2907	0.2987	0.2954	0.3019	0.1761	0.2760	0.3625	0.1749	0.2639	0.2542	0.3243	0.2803	0.0928	--	0.1910	0.3499	0.1030	0.0808
ESMJ	0.6183	0.4935	0.1845	0.4359	0.4101	0.3171	0.4703	0.5001	0.2580	0.2938	0.3999	0.5896	0.3995	0.1314	0.2522	--	0.4028	0.2386	0.2005
ESNC	0.6012	0.5520	0.3741	0.4171	0.5639	0.4680	0.5038	0.7775	0.4299	0.5218	0.3734	0.5071	0.6225	-	0.3019	0.7015	--	0.2949	0.2340
ESNI	0.4650	0.3611	0.2195	0.4775	0.4635	0.2823	0.3698	0.5045	0.3165	0.3572	0.3627	0.3335	0.3164	0.0694	0.1835	0.2243	0.5797	--	*0.0403*
ESRE	0.4914	0.3578	0.1655	0.4335	0.4554	0.2582	0.3497	0.4624	0.2900	0.4229	0.2965	0.3229	0.2582	0.0825	0.1450	0.2484	0.5697	*0.0564*	--

Reynolds genetic distances (above the diagonal), and Nei standard genetic distances (below the diagonal).
First line: 18 microsatellite loci; second line: 24 blood group and biochemical polymorphism systems
Largest distances in bold; smallest distances in italic.

[1]breed codes as in table3.
[2]DEAS DEBB DESH CZPR PLPU: 24 systems - ITMR ITNS ESMJ ESRE: 10 out of the 24 systems - ESNI: 6 out of the 24 systems.
Coefficient of variation of the Reynolds distances using the expression of table 1 and assuming d (Reynolds) = 0.025, approximately equivalent to d (Sanghvi) = 0.05.
24 BB systems: 0.28 (L = 24; k = 2.88; n = 60); 10 BB systems: 0.45 (L = 10; k = 2.73; n = 60); 6 BB systems: 0.59 (L = 6; k = 2.73; n = 60); 18 MS loci: 0.16 (L = 18; k = 10.2; n = 44).

Table 6. Marginal losses of diversity (%) based on the Weitzman diversity function.

Breed[1] loss	Reynolds distances[2]		Nei standard distances[2]	
	BB	MS	BB	MS
Individual breeds				
FRBA	-	**11.94**	-	8.65
FRBO	-	8.47	-	6.53
FRCR	-	1.31	-	1.53
FRGA	-	7.03	-	5.57
FRLI	-	9.03	-	8.06
DEAS	4.34	1.83	10.85	1.93
DEBB	6.28	4.36	16.32	4.55
DESH	6.60	6.21	6.69	**10.42**
CZPR	5.06	1.43	5.84	1.68
PLPU	8.32	3.64	11.82	3.40
ITCA	-	6.74	-	5.13
ITCT	-	6.55	-	8.71
ITCS	-	6.98	-	5.59
ITMR	**30.93**	-	**26.65**	-
ITNS	1.32	1.21	0.97	1.61
ESMJ	**21.10**	**10.56**	**19.27**	4.80
ESNC	-	10.32	-	**9.73**
ESNI	9.42	1.42	7.52	1.06
ESRE	3.75	1.12	2.45	0.98
Individual countries				
French breeds (5)	-	37.19	-	31.30
German breeds (5)	43.04	19.55	60.76	24.80
Italian breeds (2 or 4)	32.25	22.24	27.62	22.38
Spanish breeds (3 or 4)	32.98	24.97	29.23	20.36

Each column gives the reduction of the total diversity of the set of 10 (or 18) breeds when a particular breed or group of breeds is withdrawn from the set (2 largest reductions in bold).
[1] breed codes as in Table 3.
[2] BB: blood group and biochemical polymorphisms; MS: microsatellites.

5. Discussion and conclusions

This study confirms the characteristics previously established for the 2 categories of markers so far used in pigs for evaluating genetic diversity. A marked contrast exists between blood group and biochemical polymorphisms on one hand and microsatellites on the other hand, in the average number of alleles per locus, i e respectively 3 and 10 in the present sample, as well as in average heterozygosity, respectively about 0.3 and 0.5 (see table 4). Within-breed diversity however varied considerably. On an average the German and CE breeds sampled appeared to be slightly more polymorphic than the Italian and Spanish breeds for enzymes and serum proteins, though large differences in sample sizes could be partly responsible for this situation. For microsatellites, where sample sizes were more uniform, no large difference among countries appeared any more. The exceptionally low heterozygosity of the *Mora Romagnola* may be interpreted as a bottleneck effect, since the current population is known to derive from 4 founders who lived in the early 1980s.

The within-cell comparisons of distances in table 5 should be interpreted with some caution because of the unequal reliabilities of the 2 sets of markers. Applying the expression of the coefficient of variation of the distance estimation given in table 1, it can be seen that the 24 blood group and biochemical polymorphism systems allowed an estimation of distance hardly more than half as accurate as the 18 microsatellites (MS), their respective coefficients of variation being 0.28 and 0.16. The accuracy of estimation is expected to decrease with the number of systems considered and the coefficient of variation reached 0.59 in the extreme case of the distances involving ESNI which were based on only 6 systems.

This has also to be borne in mind when comparing the diversity allocations in table 6 according to the category of markers considered, or according to the distance measure chosen. However a general picture of highly unequal contributions of local breeds to the overall diversity did emerge. This confirms previous studies such as those of Laval *et al.* (2000) in pigs and of Cañon *et al.* (2001) in cattle. Table 6 should therefore provide some useful information for establishing conservation priorities, both within country and at the EU level. However, as already stressed by Laval *et al.* (2000) any conclusion that can be derived is relative to the particular sample of breeds studied. The results on a more comprehensive set of European breeds presently under investigation in the PIGBIODIV project are therefore to be awaited with interest.

The analysis of diversity in table 6 refers to the genetic relationships among breeds and does not preclude conclusions or decisions which might be based on within-breed variability. Among-population *diversity* and within-population *variability* both need to be considered in setting priorities, though the best way to combine them still needs further investigations (Barker, 2001). The question of their interrelation may also be raised. In the example discussed in the latter paper, the Weitzman diversity measure showed a low correlation with the within population allelic richness. When table 6 was compared on a breed basis to heterozygosity (or allelic richness) in table 4, a tendency appeared for the larger breed contributions to be associated with lower heterozygosities (or lower numbers of alleles), *e.g.* for *Basque*, *Mora Romagnola* and *Manchado de Jabugo*. The same tendency could also be seen in the results of Laval *et al.* (2000) and this probably reflects the important role played by genetic drift (or bottlenecks) in the genetic diversity of the European local breeds of pigs. The *Créole* pig offers the counterexample of an extremely low contribution to total diversity in spite of an extremely high allelic richness, actually the highest among the 18 breeds. Recently however, in a similar study on cattle no tendency was observed of an association between homozygosity and among-breed diversity (Cañon *et al.*, 2001). It should also be noted that the association between breed heterozygosity and contribution to between breed diversity is much weaker for BB markers than for MS markers. Though this comparison may be biased because it is based on slightly different samples of breeds, it might indicate a lesser role played by genetic drift in immunological and biochemical markers, or alternatively a higher role played by selection, as compared to microsatellites. Table 6 also suggests that the interrelation may appear more clearly with Reynolds than with Nei standard distances, since, based on the latter distance for MS, *Schwäbisch-Hällisches Schwein* and *Negro Canario* appeared as the most "unique breeds" without showing particularly low heterozygosities. It may therefore be premature to draw definite conclusions and further studies are warranted to clarify the issue.

SECTION IV

EX SITU CONSERVATION OF PIG GENETIC RESOURCES (SEMEN COLLECTIONS)

Chapter 4.1. Cryopreservation techniques for pig genetic resources conservation: a review

F. Pizzi[1], B. Pallante[2] and G. Gandini[3]

[1]*Istituto per la Difesa e la Valorizzazione del Germoplasma Animale - CNR, Via Celoria 10 – 20133 Milan, Italy*
[2]*Department of Gene Expression and Development, Roslin Institute – Roslin, Midlothian EH25 9PS, United Kingdom*
[3]*Istituto di Zootecnica, Università di Milano, Via Celoria 10 – 20133 Milan, Italy*

1. Introduction

The Convention on Biological Diversity, signed in Rio de Janeiro in 1992, lays clear guidelines for priorities among conservation strategies, including farm animal genetic resources (AnGR). The Convention identifies *in situ* conservation as the method of choice whenever possible, whilst the development of *ex situ* schemes should be considered as complement to *in situ* efforts. Within this framework, choosing the most appropriate AnGR conservation technique varies according to aims, which techniques and resources are available, species and breeding context (*e.g.* Gandini and Oldenbroek, 1999). *Ex situ* conservation can be achieved by cryopreservation of embryos, ova, semen or somatic cells. *Ex situ* live strategies include the maintenance of live animals outside their production systems, such as in natural protected areas, in experimental and show farms or in zoos.

At present conservation schemes of AnGR include the cryogenic storage of semen and embryos in gene banks as the only alternative to *in situ* or *ex situ* live. However, the development of the nuclear transfer technology might provide a new approach and the current concept of gene bank might be extended to adult somatic cells and cloned embryos.

The primary purpose of cryopreservation of AnGR is to preserve a set of genes that might be valuable in the future for breed re-establishment, creation of synthetic breeds/lines or gene introgression. Cryopreserved stocks can also be used in cryo-aided live schemes as back up if genetic problems occur, to prolong generation interval and to increase the effective size of the population (Meuwissen, 1999).

Cryopreservation compared to *in situ* schemes disregards breed evolution and maintenance of adaptive fitness. The storage of genetic materials in gene banks does not fulfil all the objectives for conservation; since it does not consider the socio-economic value of breeds neither their cultural and ecological value. Gene banks, however, can decrease the risks of *in situ* conservation schemes and should be considered as a valuable support to *in vivo* conservation. Combinations of live and cryopreservation schemes allow to achieve all conservation objectives: future economic potential, present socio-economic value, cultural and ecological value. Moreover, in these schemes the population can continue to evolve and adapt to environmental circumstances.

In cryopreservation, type of biological material, number of individuals and samples to be stored vary according to the conservation objectives. For example, if the objective is the re-establishment of a breed by using semen, the number of doses stored should allow for a sufficient number of back-cross generations in order to recover a high percentage of the genome to be re-established. Given the objectives and taking into account the success rates of the cryo-preservation technique, the material to be stored can be defined (Ollivier and Renard, 1995). However little work has been reported on type and size of samples, on related risks and costs (Brem *et al.*, 1984; Ollivier and Lauvergne, 1988; Lömker and Simon, 1994). Generally the objective is to maximise genetic variability, then the animals that contribute to the frozen stocks are chosen so that the group coancestry is minimised (Toro and Mäki-Tanila, 1999). Current technology for meiosis manipulation might provide a powerful tool to further optimise the genetic variation to be stored (Santiago and Caballero, 2000).

Samples size to be stored is generally determined according to the techniques available at the routine level. However we should consider that, at least in the controlled conditions of conservation schemes, advanced reproductive techniques such as *in vitro* fertilisation (IVF) or intracytoplasmic sperm injection (ICSI) can be expected for the very near future. In this case the full fertilisation qualities of spermatozoa and a high number of motile cells will not be anymore needed.

Reproductive technologies undergo rapid changes and improvements. This paper i.) reviews the state of the art of cryopreservation techniques in the pig species and ii.) discusses the use of current techniques and problems remaining to be solved for the conservation of pig genetic resources. In particular it analyses:

- semen cryopreservation, which has not yet achieved in the pig the efficiency observed in other species such as cattle;
- oocytes cryopreservation; particularly valuable for the preservation of endangered species;
- embryos cryopreservation, which recently started to produce results also in the pig;
- semen and embryo sexing, that might optimise cryopreservation efforts;
- nuclear transfer and cloning techniques and their possible future role in conservation.

2. Semen cryopreservation

Spermatozoa cryopreservation is today the most practical technique for storing farm animals' germplasm. Cryopreservation is less efficient in the pig than in other species, probably due some peculiar spermatozoa characteristics. Species differences in the susceptibility of sperm to cold shock are correlated with the composition of membrane lipid; resistance is greater for membranes characterised by a high degree of saturation in the phospholipid-bound fatty acid (Poulos *et al.*, 1973) and a high sterol to phospholipid ratio (Darin-Bennet and White, 1977). The plasma membrane of the boar sperm is characterised by higher protein and lower cholesterol contents when compared to other species (Parks and Lynch, 1992). The extreme cold shock sensitivity of boar semen is the greatest limiting factor to a successful freezing process. Cryopreserved boar spermatozoa have poorer motility, acrosomal integrity and viability than fresh spermatozoa. Moreover lower farrowing rate and litter size are observed when frozen semen is used.

In the seventies several techniques for deep freezing of boar semen have been developed and tested under field conditions (Pursel and Johnson 1975; Westendorf *et al.*, 1975; Paquignon and Courot 1976; Larsson *et al.*, 1977). Among the different techniques, semen has been frozen in straws (5 ml) only in the procedure developed by Westendorf *et al.* (1975), whereas all other procedures used pellets. When semen is frozen in pellets the identification of items is less easy and precise than in straws. Because storage in cryo-banks requests a high level of safety and unambiguous identification of the samples, freezing semen in pellets is not an advisable technique for gene banks.

A freezing procedure of boar semen in 0.5 ml straws was set up by Thilmant (1997). To reduce the number of straws needed for insemination dose, the spermatozoa were frozen at a high concentration (1.5×10^9 spermatozoa/ ml). With this procedure pregnancy rate and litter size achieved using frozen semen (199 inseminations) were not significantly different from those obtained with fresh semen, 79 *vs.* 80.3 % and 10.1 *vs.* 9.8 piglets respectively.

Bussière *et al.* (2000) developed a freezing method based on the use of two diluents added at different steps during the procedure. Semen was packaged in 0.5 ml straws containing

0.8 billion sperm. Double inseminations were performed using 5 straws diluted in BTS extender and only straws containing at thawing at least 30% live and normal spermatozoa were used. Pregnancy rate, measured by ultrasonography at 21 days after insemination, was 74%; a farrowing rate of 68% was recorded with a mean litter size of 9.97 (± 0.54). The interval of twenty-four hours between collection and freezing did not appear to affect semen quality. This aspect is particularly important because it suggests the possibility to collect semen directly in the farms and then transport the samples to the laboratory for freezing.

Interesting results have been recently published by Eriksson and Rodriguez-Martinez (1999; 2000b) on a new type of flat package (large plastic bags 10 x 5 cm) for frozen boar semen. The aim of this package is to provide a cheap and convenient single container during freezing, storage, thawing, reconstitution and artificial insemination. Although the results obtained through such method indicate that the deep freezing of boar semen in large bags is feasible, the problems linked to the inconvenient large size for storage represents a drawback to the use of this method for storing boar semen in cryobanks.

Frozen-thawed spermatozoa can be successfully used for *in vitro* fertilization (IVF) in pigs as demonstrated by Zheng *et al.* (1992) and Córdova *et al.* (1997). In this study frozen semen packaged in 0.25 ml straws containing 160.000 sperm has been used for *in vitro* fertilisation. The percentage of oocytes fertilised using frozen – thawed semen was 68% *vs.* 85% when fresh semen was used.

Data on Intracytoplasmatic Sperm Injection (ICSI) of *in vivo* and *in vitro* matured porcine oocytes with fresh ejaculated or frozen-thawed epididymal spermatozoa have been published by Kolbe and Holtz (1999). The spermatozoa were frozen in pellets on dry ice in a lactose-egg yolk-extender supplemented with 6% glycerol. In *in vitro*-matured oocytes injected with frozen-thawed epididymal spermatozoa, 16% showed genuine cleavage characterised by nuclear blastomeres.

Both techniques, IVF and ICSI, seem to hold considerable potential for the use of semen stored in cryobanks.

3. Oocytes cryopreservation

Cryopreservation of female germ line would be particularly valuable for the preservation of endangered breeds, though ovarian tissue and oocytes are rarely cryopreserved. Unfertilised mature oocytes are more difficult to cyopreserve than cleavage stage embryos of the same species. Many factors contribute to this difficulty, including oocyte surface to volume ratio, single membrane, temperature-sensitive metaphase spindle and zona pellucida, and susceptibility of the oocyte to chill-injury (Shaw *et al.*, 2000). On the other hand, oocytes in primordial follicles are small and tolerate cryopreservation by slow cooling very well. It is nevertheless difficult to produce mature oocytes from these primordial follicles.

Pig oocytes are damaged by short term exposure to temperature between +15° and 0°C (Didion *et al.*, 1990). The damage might be due to the high lipid content of pig oocytes since lipid removal or lipid polarization reduce chill or cryo-injury. Fatty acids content in pig oocytes was greater than in cattle and sheep oocytes (McEvoy *et al.*, 2000). Phospholipid consistently accounted for a quarter of all fatty acids in the three specie, but ruminant oocytes had a lower complement of polyunsaturates (14-19%, w/w) in this fraction than pig oocytes (34%, w/w). This species-specific difference may underlie the contrasting chilling and cryopreservation sensitivities of pig and ruminant oocytes.

4. Embryos cryopreservation

Embryos of most of livestock species can be adequately cryopreserved, with the exclusion of swine. Pig embryos suffer severe sensitivity to hypothermic conditions which limits their ability to withstand conventional cryopreservation. The survival of pig embryos may be correlated with i.) the stage of embryo development, which may be optimised *in vitro* since survival peaks during the peri-hatching blastocyst stage (Dobrinsky, 1997) and ii.) the conditions under which it develops (Pollard and Leibo, 1994).

In conventional freezing procedures a slow rate of cooling is needed to maintain the delicate balance between the various factors such as ice crystal formation, osmotic injury, toxic effect of cryoprotectants, chilling injuries, embryo fractures and alterations of intracellular organelles and cytoskeleton. An alternative method for preserving embryos is vitrification, *i.e.* the solidification of a solution (glass formation) at low temperatures without ice crystal formation. The phenomenon can be regarded as an extreme increase of viscosity and requires rapid cooling rates (2500-3000°C/min). Vitrification could be achieved by plunging sealed straws, containing the embryos, directly into liquid nitrogen (-196°C). Vitrification shows promise of eluding the danger associated with cooling sensitivity and ice crystallisation. Dobrinsky and Johnson (1994) first demonstrated the efficacy of vitrification on swine embryos where survival and subsequent development *in vitro* (around 40%) could be established in expanded and early hatched blastocyst-stage embryos.

Recently a study was conducted to document the disruption of the embryonic cytoskeleton during vitrification of pig embryos and to determine the ability of the microfilaments (MF) inhibitor cytochalasin-b to prevent irreversible disruption to MF and prevent plasma membrane disruption, while testing the developmental competence of cytoskeletal-stabilized and vitrified pig embryos (Dobrinsky *et al.*, 2000). This study showed that the pig embryos cytoskeleton could be affected by vitrification and that MF depolymerisation, prior to vitrification, improved blastocyst developmental competence after cryopreservation. Only hatched blastocysts with excellent to good morphology were transferred. A survival rate of 13% was achieved out of 224 hatched blastocysts. The authors concluded that vitrified embryos can produce live, healthy piglets that grow normally and when mature have excellent fecundity. Vitrification of hatched blastocysts seems to be a viable method for long term preservation of pig embryos and a useful tool to preserve genetic resources in gene banks especially when the objective of the bank is the re-establishment of a breed.

The ultra-rapid cooling OPS (Open Pullet Straw) method was tested for its ability to preserve embryos from chilling damage (Vajta *et al.*, 1997). The technology involves the freezing of unhatched blastocysts in a specially designed narrow straw containing a very small volume of cryoprotectant (2μl), plunged directly into liquid nitrogen. Berthelot *et al.* (2000) have tested this ultra rapid freezing method for vitrification of pig embryos aged 5-6 days recovered from Meishan and Large White gilts. The ability of embryos to develop after cryopreservation was evaluated either by *in vitro* culture for 1 to 5 days to record the number of hatched blastocysts, or by surgical transfer in gilts. A survival rate of nearly 10% was achieved out of 400 unhatched blastocysts transferred The authors conclude that OPS allows cryopreservation of unhatched porcine blastocysts.

5. Semen and embryo sexing

Predetermining the sex of offspring has been for a long time a goal of livestock producers. Sex pre-selection provides an opportunity to improve the efficiency of cryopreservation in conservation schemes. It allows to store only sperm needed to produce offspring of the desired sex. In backcrossing for breed re-establishment only female offspring is required and sexed semen will reduce consistently costs and time of reconstruction. Sex pre-selection can also be of use in the creation of synthetic breeds/lines, gene introgression and cryo-aided live schemes. This is particularly true in uniparous species, but it can be advantageous also in the pig.

Various methods have been developed and tested for sexing semen. Most of them have been devised on the basis of supposed differences between X and Y spermatozoa, such as size, motility, surface charge, sperm surface antigens or specific proteins.

A sexing technology based on the differential amount of DNA present in X- and Y-chromosome bearing sperm was developed by Johnson and co-workers since 1989. Relative DNA content is determined by quantitative staining with a fluorochrome (Hoechst 33342). The difference in DNA amount in X and Y bearing sperm varies according to the species; pigs carry about 3.6% percent more DNA in their X sperm than in their Y sperm, cattle 3.8% more and humans 2.8%. A modified flow cytometry sorting has been used to sort X and Y bearing sperm. In pigs offspring have been born as a result of using gender-selected sperm for surgical intratubal insemination (Rath et al., 1994), IVF of in vivo matured oocytes (Rath et al., 1997) and IVF of IVM oocytes (Abeydeera et al., 1998; Rath et al., 1999). Even if the sorting speed has been increased from 350.000 sperm/hour of the original technology to 11 million sperm/hour (Johnson and Welch, 1999), further improvements are needed before the technology can be routinely used. Pig insemination requires a large number of sperm and thus a much longer time to sort the specific semen population. In this regard, the use of deep artificial insemination with a low sperm dose would be advantageous (Johnson et al., 2000a).

Recently, sorted boar sperm has been successfully frozen. The frozen-thawed semen was used for surgical insemination. Viability assessments, based on motility estimates, demonstrated that about 30% of the sperm could survive both sorting and freezing. Very preliminary results with frozen sorted boar sperm has produced embryos and healthy piglets (Johnson et al., 2000b).

A new sexing approach based on immunology has been developed (Blecher et al., 1999). This approach seems highly valuable since it offers hope for inexpensive batch processing for sexing sperm. Moreover the immunologically based system would be minimally invasive. The method is based on the hypotheses that sex chromosomes control the expression of X- and Y-sex-chromosome-specific proteins (X- or Y-SCSPs) which are present on the surface of sperm cells and that cell sex-specific proteins are more highly conserved than non-sex-specific proteins. The process shows some promise but its efficacy has not yet been fully tested. No data have been published on the use of this technology in the pig but some experiments are in course.

Sexing embryos prior to transfer using PCR is routinely available in cattle. Concerning pig Kawarasaki et al. (2000) have recently demonstrated that embryos at the >32-cell stage can be sexed within 2 hours from collection using the Fluorescence In Situ Hybridisation (FISH) method. Such rapid diagnosis enables embryos sexed to develop into normal piglets. However in order to establish that FISH sexing is effective for controlling the sex in pigs additional embryo transfers would be needed and the viability of the sexed embryos verified.

6. Somatic cell nuclear transfer

A paper published in Nature in February 1996 (Campbell et al., 1996) reporting the cloning of two lambs from foetal somatic (body) cells by researchers of the Roslin Institute provided the first evidence in mammals of the reversibility of DNA quiescence. A further breakthrough was represented by the birth of a lamb (Wilmut et al., 1997), named Dolly, cloned by researchers from the same Institute using somatic cells isolated from the mammary gland of an ewe. This pioneer work proved that differentiation is a reversible process since nuclei from differentiated cells, after transfer to a recipient oocyte, can be reprogrammed to initiate and complete embryonic development giving rise to all the cell types, organised in tissues and organs, present in an organism at the end of embryogenesis.

The cell cloning or nuclear transfer (NT) technique involves the removal of genetic material from a mature oocyte or a zygote and its replacement with genetic material of a donor cell. There are currently two main variants of the nuclear transfer technique. The first variant was developed in sheep by researchers at the Roslin Institute and was used to clone Dolly (Wilmut et al., 1997). With this procedure whole somatic cells, made quiescent by culture with low serum concentrations, are used as donors. After placing them in the perivitelline space of enucleated oocytes, the cells are fused to the recipient oocyte using an electric current (electro-fusion). The electric pulses also induce the release of calcium from the eggs' internal stores, the same signal triggered by sperm at fertilization, and lead to cell cycle resumption in the reconstructed embryo (activation). Therefore, in this system, fusion and activation occur simultaneously. A second variant of the NT technique (Wakayama et al.,1998) was developed in mice by researchers in Hawaii (Honolulu technique). With this procedure freshly isolated cells, already in a quiescent state, are used as donors. Donor cells are stripped of the cytoplasm by suction into a piezo-electrically controlled micropipette, and only the nucleus is injected into the cytoplasm of recipient oocyte. Activation is induced 1-6 hours after fusion (delayed activation) by culturing the reconstructed embryos in medium containing strontium. The removal of the cell cytoplasm and the delay between fusion and activation are thought to enhance nuclear reprogramming after transfer to the recipient oocyte. In both techniques the reconstructed embryos are then cultured and transferred to surrogate recipients for development to term.

After Dolly's birth live offspring have been produced by somatic NT (for review see Colman, 2000) in a variety of species. Development to term has been obtained from foetal somatic cells in cattle, goats, sheep, mice and cows. Cattle, mice and pigs have also been produced from adult cell donors. All cloned animals appear to be healthy and sheep (Shiels et al., 1999), mice (Wakayama et al., 1998) and cattle (unpublished data) clones have also proved fertile. Albeit these encouraging results, the main problem of NT still remains its very poor efficiency in terms of post-implantation development and postnatal survival. These problems seem to stem from an incomplete and/or incorrect reprogramming of the donor nucleus after NT. Some of the biological factors influencing the remodelling of the donor chromatin (Sun and Moor, 1995) have already been identified and are: the cell cycle stage of the donor cell; the developmental stage of the recipient oocyte; the relative cell cycle stage of the donor nucleus and recipient oocyte. The efficiency of NT is expected to improve greatly in the short-, medium-term as researchers acquire a better understanding of the reprogramming process.

A lot of efforts have been put in the development of the cloning technology in pigs. This interest has been fuelled by the possibility of producing transgenic pigs by combining the cloning technology with the gene targeting technology (Polejaeva and Campbell, 2000) to produce animals for xenotransplantation (Persidis, 1999). The market for solid organs alone could be worth 6bn euros, with as much again from cellular therapies, such as transplantation of pancreatic islets in diabetic patients.

Despite all these efforts the cloning of pigs has proved more difficult than other mammals mainly due to technical difficulties (Prather et al., 1999). The first pig cloning experiments were carried in the late 80's. However, until recently, there was only one report about the successful cloning of a piglet using a blastomere from an early embryo as donor of genetic material (Prather et al., 1989). A major breakthrough in pig cloning occurred when 5 piglets were cloned by using granulosa cells as donors (Polejaeva et al., 2000). Development to term was also obtained in two separate studies using foetal fibroblasts as donor cells (Onishi et al.,

2000; Betthauser et al., 2000). These data prove that somatic cloning of pigs is indeed possible, though less efficiently than in other livestock species, and suggests that in the future this technology could be used in conservation programmes. Other reports about the successful cloning of porcine embryos using cryopreserved blastomeres (Nagashima et al., 1997) also suggest that the cryopreservation of pig cells does not affect their ability to support development to term of reconstructed embryos.

Pig cloning raises for both technical and biological problems. The main technical disadvantage is represented by the fragility of the porcine egg, that can be easily damaged and lysed during micromanipulation at the time of enucleation and fusion. In addition the high lipid content of pig oocytes makes it difficult to visualise the metaphase plate and the polar body during enucleation. This leads to an increase of the time of exposure to UV light (short-wavelength, high energy light), detrimental for the oocyte but necessary to excite the fluorochromes used to stain the DNA localised in the oocyte metaphase plate and in the polar body. These problems might be overcome by the development of techniques aimed at reducing mechanical and physical insults associated with NT. The application to pig cloning of technical advances such as chemical enucleation (Baguisi and Overström, 2000), use of long-wavelength (low energy) DNA dyes and virus mediated fusion (Dominko et al., 1999) is therefore expected to increase the efficiency of NT in pigs in the near future. Activation is also known to be less efficient in pig than in other mammalian species. However more efficient protocols are currently being developed (Macháty et al., 1999). The low efficiency of pig cloning might also result from the early shift, in this species, from maternal to embryonic control of transcription (Telford et al., 1990), when Zygote Genome Activation (ZGA) takes place. This occurs at the 4-cell stage, in pig, at the 8-cell stage in cattle and rabbit, and at the 8-, 16-cell stage in sheep. As a result of this, the donor cell nucleus, after transfer to the recipient oocyte, has very little time to be reprogrammed and to become able to direct embryo development. Therefore pig cloning will benefit greatly from basic research aimed at understanding the factors influencing the efficiency of donor nucleus reprogramming. This is also suggested by the fact that recently cloned pigs were obtained from adult cells by using the re-cloning technique(Polejaeva et al., 2000), which is thought to enhance nuclear reprogramming (Zakhartchenko et al., 1999).

7. Cloning and conservation

The cryopreservation programmes reported in both EAAP and FAO animal genetic resources data banks (see URLs in Appendix to chapter 1.1) refer to storage of semen and embryos. Both techniques are time consuming, costly and technically demanding: 1) donor animals have to be adult and fertile; 2) donor animals should be transported to well equipped facilities, both for health and technical reasons; 3) collection, processing and cryopreservation of semen and embryos require highly skilled personnel; 4) biological samples must be processed and stored promptly (hours) in liquid nitrogen, once thawed they must be immediately used; 5) in case of storage failure semen and embryos are damaged.

The development of the NT technology might provide a more practical approach (Woolliams and Wilmut, 1999). The use of cloning, as opposed to semen and embryo cryopreservation, would have several advantages: 1) sub-adult or infertile animals can be used as donors; 2) biological samples (blood, skin biopsies, hair follicles) would be collected directly on farm and then transported to central laboratories for further processing; 3) collection would be quick and would require relatively low expertise; 4) in central laboratories samples would be placed in temporary cultures and frozen following simple protocols, all over a period of days; 5) in case of storage failure, cells could be thawed, sub-cultured and stored again.

Donor cells of choice for cloning of endangered breeds should be somatic cells. Foetal cells might be more successful than adult cells in cloning, however the mother must be sacrificed. The cell type of choice should have the following characteristics: easy accessibility, lack of invasiveness even with repetitive collections, no limitations on animal sex or age. Not all cell types that have been successfully used for adult somatic cloning have these features, the main limitation being their exclusive male (Sertoli cells) or female (cumulus cells, granulosa cells, mammary gland cells, oviductal cells) origin (for review see Colman, 2000). Lymphocytes, isolated from blood samples, (Galli *et al.*, 1999) and adult fibroblasts and epithelial cells (Wakayama and Yanagimachi, 1999; Kubota *et al.*, 2000; Ogura *et al.*, 2000b), isolated from skin biopsies or plucked hair, might be the best candidates. These cell types can be easily isolated in both sexes using routine procedures well established in all farm animals. The storage of hair follicles, skin biopsies and blood samples for future cloning of endangered species has also been suggested in a recent FAO workshop (FAO, 1998a).

In some cases, isolation of cells from old animals might be desirable, as they often carry important genetic variation. Recent reports suggest that the age of the donor animal does not affect NT success (Wells *et al.*, 1998a; Kubota *et al.*, 2000) and that cultured cell senescence might even improve the development of the reconstructed embryos. Skin fibroblasts isolated from an 17 years old bull and granulosa cells isolated from a 13 year old heifer (Wells *et al.*, 1998a) were able to support development to term.

Long term storage in liquid nitrogen does not seem to affect the ability of somatic cells to support development of cloned embryos. Offspring have been produced from cryopreserved cattle lymphocytes (Galli *et al.*, 1999) and mouse Sertoli cells (Ogura *et al.*, 2000a). In cattle (Yang *et al.*, 1993; Peura *et al.*, 1999) and pig (Nagashima *et al.*, 1997) nuclei from cryopreserved or vitrified blastomeres, after transfer to recipient oocytes, were still able to support development to blastocyst stage, in some cases with efficiencies similar to fresh embryos (Peura *et al.*, 1999). These results are important since cloned embryos could be cryopreserved and blastomeres used later for embryo multiplication through a second round of embryonic cloning (re-cloning; Peura and Trounson, 1999).

A suitable source of recipient oocytes should also be considered. For conservation purposes females from another breed might be the only option when i) the breed has gone extinct and no oocytes or embryos are available, or ii) the female population is particularly small or it is difficult to handle the animals for oocyte collection. Moreover, cloning is still a very inefficient technology, in particular in the pig, the main problem being the low percentages of development to term and low survival to adulthood. This might generate the need for a large number of oocytes which could only be obtained from other breeds.

The use of oocytes from another breed implies that the latter will also be the source of the cytoplasmic DNA present. Recent reports (Evans *et al.*, 1999; Takeda *et al.*, 1999) clearly show that in cloned embryos, just like in fertilized eggs, inheritance of mitochondrial DNA (mtDNA) is, in most cases, strictly maternal. Reconstructed embryos receive a type of mtDNA from the donor cell and one from the recipient oocyte, therefore they are heteroplasmic for mtDNA during early development. Nevertheless, as they reach the blastocyst stage, they become homoplasmic, retaining only the oocyte genotype for mtDNA. Cloned offspring are also homoplasmic and express in all their tissues only the mtDNA derived from the recipient oocyte. At present there is little evidence that mtDNA is a major component of genetic variation for important traits, a situation possibly due to the difficulties of detecting mitochondrial variation in quantitative traits (Gibson *et al.*, 1997). However reports on the relationship between mtDNA mutations and phenotypic expressions, such as disease (Wallace, 1992) and ageing (Soong *et al.*, 1992) in humans and milk production (Schutz *et al.*, 1994) and carcass traits (Mannen *et al.*, 1998) in cattle, suggest that there might be interactions between mtDNA and nuclear genome which might affect the outcome of "interbreed" cloning.

To prevent genetic contamination with mtDNA of another breed, cryopreservation of oocytes or ovarian sections from endangered breeds should be considered. In recent years there has been a breakthrough in female gamete cryopreservation and there have been now a few reports about cryopreserved oocytes supporting development to term of IVF, ICSI (Tucker *et al.,* 1998; Kubota *et al.,* 1998; Sztein *et al.,* 2000), or even cloned embryos (Kubota *et al.,* 1998). Future research leading to an increase in NT efficiency may reduce dramatically the number of oocytes needed in cloning experiments. Therefore preventive cryo-storage of oocytes or ovarian tissue sections from rare breeds should be carried out, whenever possible.

The recent developments in cloning suggest that cryobanking of somatic cells is a concrete possibility and it should be integrated into AnGR conservation schemes, especially for those species/breeds where gamete banking is not feasible or in those countries were cryopreservation is not an option due to technical difficulties. Cloning for conservation purposes has already been successfully used to preserve the last surviving cow of the Enderby Island cattle breed from New Zealand (Wells *et al.,* 1998a) and the Argali (*Ovis ammon*) sheep from Asia (White *et al.,* 1999). Zoological parks are already taking into consideration cloning strategies to maintain genetic diversity of their captive populations of wild endangered species (Ryder and Benirschle, 1997; Wildt, 1992). Finally, also FAO has acknowledged the potential of cloning for *ex situ* conservation and has suggested guidelines for its implementation in conservation programmes (FAO, 1998a).

At present there are still some limitations to the use of cloning for conservation purposes. The main problem is the low efficiency of the NT technology (Colman, 2000). Although pre-implantation development (blastocyst stage) does not seem to be a problem in most mammals (20% sheep, 40% mice, 20% cattle) with the only exception of pigs (1%-5.3%), post-implantation development (7.5%-8%sheep; 1.1%-6.7% mice; 9%-14 % cattle) is very low. Foetal loss is usually associated with the Large Offspring Syndrome (LOS; Young *et al.,* 1998) characterised by oversized foetuses and placentas. These abnormalities are suspected to stem from incomplete nuclear reprogramming of the donor cell after transfer to the recipient oocyte. Further losses occur after birth (33%-61% sheep; 25%-50% cattle), often associated with respiratory failure and with immune system abnormalities (sheep, Wells *et al.,* 1998b; Wilmut *et al.,* 1997; cattle, Wells *et al.,* 1998a; Cibelli *et al.,* 1998; Renard *et al.,* 1999), which might be caused by abnormal developmental gene expression. A better understanding of the biological factors responsible for the correct and complete reprogramming of the donor nuclei is therefore essential.

Cloned animals must be healthy, fertile and show good fitness. The report that Dolly's telomeres were significantly shorter than in sheep of the same age group (Shiels *et al.,* 1999) suggested that cloning might affect the health and life expectancy of cloned animals. Telomeres are DNA sequences located at the end of chromosomes and their shortening is associated with cell senescence (Greider, 1996; King, 1999), therefore it was thought that clones might have a shorter life-span. Further evidence failed to confirm this hypothesis. Up to date all the animals cloned by NT appear to be phenotypically normal, with no signs of premature ageing. Fertility of cloned animals also appears to be unaffected as several sheep, mice and cattle produced from NT experiments (sheep, Wilmut *et al.,* 1997; Wells *et al.,* 1998b; mice, Wakayama *et al.,* 1999; Ogura *et al.,* 2000a; cattle, unpublished data) have produced healthy offspring. Some of these offspring (mice) have also proven fertile.

Finally, before cloning is integrated into conservation programmes, procedures for testing the health status of donor animals and of the biological material collected need to be defined. Requirements for somatic cells might be simpler than those currently used for semen and embryos storage (FAO, 1998b), although aspects such as latent viruses deserve some attention.

Chapter 4.2. Pig semen banks in Europe

F. Labroue[1], M. Luquet[1], P. Guillouet[2], J.F. Bussière[2], P. Glodek[3], W. Wemheuer[3], G. Gandini[4], F. Pizzi[4], J.V. Delgado[5], A. Poto[6], B. Peinado[6], J.R.B. Sereno[5] and L. Ollivier[7]

[1]*I.T.P., Pôle Amélioration de l'Animal, BP 3, 35651 Le Rheu Cedex, France*
[2]*I.N.R.A., Unité Expérimentale d'Insémination Caprine et Porcine, 86480 Rouillé, France*
[3]*Université de Göttingen, Albrecht-Thaer Weg 3 - 37075 Göttingen, Germany*
[4]*IDVGA-CNR, Via Celoria 10 - 20133 Milano, Italy*
[5]*Departamento de Genética, Universitad de Cordoba, Avenida Medina Azahara 9 - 14005 Cordoba, Spain*
[6]*Centro de Investigacion y Desarollo Agroalimentaria – 30150 La Alberca, Murcia, Spain*
[7]*I.N.R.A., Station de Génétique Quantitative et appliquée, 78352 Jouy-en-Josas Cedex, France*

1. Introduction

Conservation of animal genetic resources, as an insurance against the risks of genetic erosion, can be achieved through live animal preservation (*in situ* programme), or through cryopreservation of semen or embryos (*ex situ* programme). In pigs, *ex situ* conservation programmes are still very few (see chapter 1.1). The cryopreservation techniques available, as well as their expected evolution in the future, are reviewed in chapter 4.1. Deep freezing of semen is presently the only operational means sufficiently reliable for storing pig germplasm, and this technique has indeed been successfully used in breeding practice in Europe for the last 25 years. In this chapter, we will present the design and requirements to be met for achieving a most secure long-term storage of a breed germplasm, as well as the costs implied. The present situation of pig gene banks in the 4 countries participating in the RESGEN12 project will also be reviewed.

2. The objectives of a rational cryopreservation using semen banks

Cryopreservation (in liquid nitrogen at –195°C) of semen or embryos is a method of *ex situ* conservation of animal genetic resources, which can complement live or *in situ* conservation (see chapter 4.1). The costs of the different methods of conservation in farm animals have been evaluated for the first time by Smith (1984). More recent evaluations in different countries have been reviewed by Ollivier and Renard (1995). In this paper, security constraints applying to the collections stored were emphasised, implying that semen or embryos be stored at several locations, say two at least. The quantities stored at one location should then permit to renew the stock accidentally lost at the other. When only semen is stored, the renewal should be made possible in the extreme situation of a breed extinct, in which case no breeding female is available. In this case, it will be necessary to grade up any female population available with the remaining semen, through a back-crossing system on a sufficient number of generations. This is particularly the case in pigs, when embryo conservation is not yet operational in practice.

A sufficient number of semen doses to allow re-establishing an extinct breed should therefore be stored in each of at least two different locations. The evaluation of the number of doses needed in cattle has been explained by Lömker and Simon (1994). Ollivier and Renard (1995) have extended the method to various farm animal species, and expressed the number of doses needed as a function of the breeding scheme applied, namely the number of generations, the generation interval and the reproduction parameters of the species considered. In pigs, we assume that only gilts are used at each generation, in order to obtain one generation per year. One can then evaluate the total number F of gilts to be inseminated given a number n of generations in the grading-up process, such as generation 1 is made of the initial group of purebred females, generation 2 is the F_1, generation 3 is the first back-cross (BC_1), and so on until generation n which is BC_{n-2}. The nth generation carries a proportion $1- (0.5)^{n-1}$ of the genes in the panel of frozen semen. With an objective of N fertile gilts at generation n, the total number of gilts to be inseminated (including the N gilts of generation n) is the sum of the n terms of a geometrical progression, such as $F = N (1 + r+ r^2+...+ r^{n-1}) = N (r^n-1)/(r-1)$, in which the ratio r is the expected number of inseminations needed to obtain one fertile daughter. This ratio is thus the inverse of the number (f) of fertile daughters expected per insemination. If d doses are needed per insemination, the total number of doses (D) to be stored per breed in each location is given by:

$$D = dN(r^n - 1)/(r-1) \qquad (1)$$

Equation (1) assumes r different from 1 and reduces to $D = d N n$ when $r = 1$. It should also be noted that D includes the number of doses needed to inseminate the N gilts of generation n, which would not be needed if the males and females of the last generation were intercrossed.

Table 1 shows how D varies according to n (from 4 to 7)and f (at most equal to one), assuming double-dose insemination ($d = 2$) and an objective of 25 fertile females in the nth generation ($N = 25$). The particular case when the expected number f of fertile daughters per insemination exceeds one, i.e. $r < 1$, will be discussed below. The table also shows the percentage of the genome retrieved at the end of the operation, as well as its lower limit at $P = 0.95$, as derived by Hill (1993). It can be seen that the variance of the percentage retrieved decreases as n increases. The number of doses needed increases rapidly with n. In fact, the increase is exponential when $r > 1$, and linear when $r = 1$.

Table 1. Number of AI doses required in each conservation site in order to re-establish a breed through a repeated back-crossing scheme (numbers rounded to the upper ten) by applying equation (1) in text.

	Number of generations (n)			
	4	5	6	7
Percentage of conserved genome recovered at generation n				
average ($1-0.5^{n-1}$)	0.88	0.94	0.97	0.98
lower limit at P=0.95	0.82	0.90	0.94	0.97
Number of fertile daughters per AI double dose (f)				
2/3	410	660	1040	1610
0.75	330	490	700	980
0.90	240	320	400	500
1	200	250	300	350

Another constraint in setting up a gene bank relates to the genetic variability of the sample of boars being collected. Following Smith (1984), the minimum number of males to be retained is usually 25, in order to obtain a maximum increase of 2% inbreeding when re-establishing the breed. It is worth noting that 25 is the recommended number of males able to produce good quality semen after thawing, which requires collecting about 30 boars. On the basis of this recommendation, it can be seen that the number of doses to be stored per boar may vary from 8 (200/25) to 65 (1610/25) according to the values retained for n and f in table 1.

As to the number N of breeding females, it should be noted that the initial genetic variability is best maintained when all males are used in each generation. This implies that N should at least be equal to the number of males cryopreserved, that at least N females be inseminated in each generation, and, consequently, that the number of doses should not be less than $d\,N\,n$, the value corresponding to one fertile daughter obtained per insemination, *i.e.* $f = 1$. It can easily be seen that when $f > 1$ a breed might indeed be re-established using a very limited number of females in the first generation cross. For instance, assuming $f = 2$, only 4 females would be needed initially in order to obtain 25 females in the 4th generation, and only one female when $n = 6$ or more, if this constraint of 25 males mated to 25 different females in each generation were disregarded.

3. The semen freezing techniques and their evolution

The cryopreservation of boar semen at low temperature has been intensively investigated since the early 70s (Polge *et al.,* 1970), and reviewed in chapter 4.1 of this book. Until recently, fertility and prolifically results have remained unsatisfactory. As an example, a field experiment on the use of frozen semen after a decade of conservation at INRA-SEIA of Rouillé (Vienne) only yielded an average of 2.3 piglets born per dose of frozen semen (Ollivier *et al.,* 1991). Based on those results, and taking into account mortality and fertility of the female progeny, a value of f below 1 had to be assumed. The recommendations of the French Ministry of Agriculture, also retained in this RESGEN12 project, were indeed to take $f = 2/3$ and $n = 6$, which led to recommend 80 doses per boar, in order to reach the 2000 doses (80×25) needed to accommodate the two sites of conservation (see Table 1).

New freezing procedures of boar semen in 0.5 ml straws now allow to achieve pregnancy rate and litter size approaching the values obtained with fresh semen (see chapter 4.1). Depending on further confirmation of these results, it can therefore be envisaged to lower the requirements in number of doses per boar and to assume that one fertile daughter per double dose could be guaranteed in the future. The recent recommendations of an expert group convened by FAO (FAO-UNEP, 1998b) were based on the latter assumption. However, the number of doses recommended per breed is close to 4000 (20 boars $\times$ 1235 straws/6 straws per dose), well above the figures of Table 1 for $f = 0.67$. The reason for this difference appears to be the wider range of objectives assigned to the cryoconserved material in the FAO report. Additional goals mentioned there include creation of new breeds, support for *in vivo* conservation and research on gene effects.

Table 2 presents an evaluation of the costs of creating a collection of boar semen for the strict purpose of *ex situ* conservation, and also the annual costs of storage, according to the option taken as to the number of doses per boar. It should be noted that the costs of training the boars may exceed the amount assumed here, since considerable variation exists among individuals in the time needed, and also because the training of boars not retained for collection is not considered. On the basis of 2000 doses (80×25) for conserving a breed, it can be seen that the cost of a breed collection is near 30 000 euros, while the annual storage cost represents less than 1% of this amount.

Table 2. Costs per boar (in euros) of a pig gene bank made of two conservation sites (excluding facilities and heavy equipment).

	80 doses per boar 400 straws[1] 12 collections 90 days of presence[2]	40 doses per boar 200 straws[1] 6 collections 60 days of presence[2]	20 doses per boar 100 straws[1] 3 collections 50 days of presence[2]
Fixed costs per boar			
Boar price	305	305	305
Transportation, veterinary costs and consumables	524	524	524
Variable costs			
Housing, feeding, labour	322	215	169
Small equipment	13	7	3
Total collection cost per boar	1164	1051	1001
Total cost of storage per boar	10	5	2.5

[1]A dose is made up of 5 0.5ml straws, each straw containing 8×10^8 spermatozoa (two doses are usually needed per insemination).
[2]A training period of one month is assumed.

4. The situation of pig cryopreservation in France

Storage of frozen semen for conservation purposes, started as early as 1982, using the pellet technique of Paquignon *et al.* (1986). From 1982 to 1986, 18 boars were first collected at the INRA centre of Nouzilly (Indre-et-Loire). Then from 1987 to 1995, 43 boars were collected at the INRA-SEIA of Rouillé (Vienne). The 61 boars collected were distributed among the 5 French local breeds as follows: 12 *Basque* (BA), 14 *Gascon* (GA), 13 *Blanc de l'Ouest* (BO), 15 *Limousin* (LI) and 7 *Bayeux* (BY). This first step led to a total of 1416 doses stored. The number of doses per boar was much below 80, as it varied between 9 and 41, with an average of 23 doses per boar. Since the beginning of the RESGEN12 project, further semen collection and freezing were carried out using 0.5 ml straws, as described by Bussière *et al.* (2000), with an objective of 80 doses per boar. Up to 1998, 18 additional boars were collected allowing to store 1440 supplementary doses, distributed among 15 BA, 2 LI, and 1 BY boars. From 1998 to 2000, 13 BY, 18 GA, 15 LI and 16 BO boars have been collected.

In 1998, it was decided to share the stock of pellets initiated in 1982 between a national primary site of conservation ACSEDIATE, located at Maisons-Alfort (Val de Marne) and SEIA, acting as a secondary site of conservation. A stock of 547 doses was then transferred from SEIA to ACSEDIATE. The same procedure has later been implemented for the straws prepared from 1998 on during the RESGEN12 project. The present situation of the French pig gene bank is summarised in Table 3, showing about 7 000 doses stored from 135 boars, originating themselves from 130 different sires.

Table 3. Present state (end of 2000) of the French pig gene bank.

	Breed					
	Basque	*Bayeux*	*Gascon*	*Limousin*	*Blanc de l'Ouest*	*Total*
Primary site						
nb of boars	27	8	12	14	11	72
nb of doses in pellets[1]	114	68	121	126	118	547
nb of doses in straws[2]	720	51	0	90	0	861
total nb of doses	834	119	121	216	118	1408
Secondary site						
nb of boars	27	20	28	30	30	135
nb of doses in pellets[1]	169	121	190	194	195	869
nb of doses in straws[2]	600	944	1120	1032	1190	4886
total nb of doses	769	1065	1310	1226	1385	5755
Total number of doses	1603	1184	1431	1442	1503	7163
Total number of boars	27	20	28	30	30	135
Total number of sires of boars	26	18	28	29	29	130

[1]Dose = 0.6×10^{8} spermatozoa
[2]Dose defined in table 2

5. The situation of pig cryopreservation in Germany

In the framework of RESGEN12, a semen bank was established at the Veterinary Institute of Göttingen University, which contained the frozen semen doses of each boar included in the programme. It is intended to allocate half of the doses of each boar to two State Ministries of Agriculture (namely Niedersachsen, where a BB conservation project is financed and Baden-Württemberg, where the SH conservation is sponsored) for long term storage and administration. The individual boars with their parental pedigree and total number of semen doses frozen are given in table 4 for Saddlebacks (AS/DS, SH) and in table 5 for *Bunte Bentheimer* (BB).

In Saddlebacks 19 AS/DS boars from 6 sire lines (12 sublines) are stored which represent all but one presently still available sire lines of the breed and thereby characterise the within breed genetic diversity very well. All Saddleback boars in the semen reserve have undergone an MHS-test for the halothane gene and were found to be homozygous normal (NN-genotype).

The BB lines originated from six different foundation sires, of which two were lost in the first years of the conservation project because no sons of them were kept. But in the pedigrees of two very old breeding sows (730 and 737) these two boars were detected and therefore these two sows were taken as founders of separated lines F1 (going back to founder boar 800) and F2 (going back to founder boar 801). Although 11 of the boars came from the dominating H sire line it has been tried to cover as many son-grandson-families as possible, and therefore the whole family spectrum of the BB population from 1997/98 was represented in the semen reserve. In contrast, in the live population not all lines have survived the two low price years in which 5 out of 7 herds were discontinued.

Table 4. Frozen semen reserve of German Saddlebacks (AS/DS and SH).

No.	Boar No[1]	Breed/Line[2]		Sire	Dam	Sire of dam	Total no. doses[3]
1	3	AS/DS	G1	29152	28410	29147	213
2	6	"	"	"	28295	2671	302
3	68	"	G2	60015	60250	60012	200
4	802906	"	G3	MV 671	MV 010	30574700	52 (AI)
5	58	"	H1	40119	41367	40076	154
6	31604/10	"	H2	803023	31604	60010	105 (AI)
7	4	"	O1	29174	28298	40100	181
8	5	"	"	"	28254	2657	217
9	7	"	O2	40156	41451	NHB	212
10	8	"	"	"	41452	NHB	150
11	79	"	P1	40116	41403	40073	198
12	80	"	"	"	41404	"	206
13	82	"	P2	60003	60243	60001	126
14	1	"	P2	"	"	"	120
15	77	"	S1	60010	60258	60003	203
16	803021	"	"	"	9434	60002	76 (AI)
17	2	"	V1	60019	60046	60010	188
18	59	"	V2	40093	41391	40081	245
19	60	"	"	"	"	"	234
20	11	SH	GO1	604	1424	501	208
21	13	"	"	"	1627	226	37
22	15	"	GO2	605	1517	703	157
23	18	"	HE1	503	1327	220	173
24	14	"	HE2	506	1629	226	169
25	12	"	HE3	507	1686	224	145
26	16	"	HS	703	1511	603	227
27	9	"	R1	226	1425	501	85
28	10	"	"	"	1623	"	153
Total			10	19	26	21	4736

[1]Boar No = register number of the boar in semen reserve; [2]Breed/Line = Saddleback population AS/DS /sire line; [3]Total number of doses (as defined in table 2), which will be equally divided between two storage locations; AI = semen samples from AI-boars.

Table 5. Frozen semen reserve of Bunte Bentheimer.

No.	Boar No.	MHS test[1]	Line	Sire	Dam	Sire of dam	Total no. doses[2]
1	83	NP	H1	961	951	844	175
2	25	NN	"	"	949	838	146
3	26	NP	"	"	992	844	143
4	65	NP	H2	963	791	32258	135
5	67	NP	"	"	728	32182	148
6	86	NP	H3	33112	916	32409	125
7	89	NP	"	"	917	"	193
8	87	NP	H4	844	949	838	129
9	88	NP	"	"	"	"	148
10	63	NN	H5	846	912	32258	171
11	64	PP	"	"	929	836	133
12	84	NP	KA	33099	954	828	116
13	19	NN	KU	33113	930	836	187
14	20	NN	"	"	776	32258	228
15	21	NN	"	"	912	"	168
16	22	NN	"	"	"	"	173
17	69	NN	S1	850	907	826	313
18	70	NN	"	"	"	"	231
19	24	NN	"	"	919	32567	183
20	23	NP	S2	1009(69)	998	961	167
21	27	NP	(F1)[3]	995(70)	737	32258	291
22	28	NP	(F2)[3]	33113	730	32182	149
Total	22	0.30 P	6	10	17	10	3 852

[1]Halothane genotype (NN homozygous normal, NP heterozygous, PP homozygous for the susceptibility gene); [2]total number of doses (as defined in table 2), which will be equally divided between two storage locations; [3](F1, F2) subline (see text).

6. The situation of pig cryopreservation in Italy

A programme of *ex situ* conservation was initiated within the framework of RESGEN12 in the four breeds *Cinta Senese* (CS), *Casertana* (CT), *Mora Romagnola* (MR) and *Nera Siciliana* (NS). The semen bank was developed in partnership with the private AI company ELPZOO, located at Zorlesco, Lodi. This is the first case in Italy where a private company supports consistently a programme of conservation of farm animal genetic resources.

The primary site of storage of the bank will be at ELPZOO. Secondary sites will be: (i) ANAS (national association of pig breeders) for the *Cinta Senese*, *Mora Romagnola* and *Nera Siciliana* breeds, (ii) ConSDABI Institute, near Benevento, for the *Casertana* breed. Discussion has been started to define the future management of the pig semen bank: the bank will be donated to the Ministry of Agriculture Politics, in accordance with the guidelines of the Convention on Biological Diversity (Rio de Janeiro, 1992), and it will be managed by a consortium including scientific institutions, breeders' associations and the national administration, according to rules of access to be defined.

The major difficulties encountered in the creation of the semen bank were: (i) to collect boars widely dispersed over small herds, (ii) to find unrelated animals (in most of the breeds, due to small population size, mean relationship is very high), (iii) health regulations applying to AI Centres, which are difficult to be met in free-ranging farming systems, (iv) the long training period of boars and the low percentage of animals producing semen, particularly in those animals coming from free-ranging farming systems.

By the end of the project, 3800 doses were stored, and distributed over the four breeds, CT CS, MR and NS, as shown in Table 6.

Table 6. Present state (end of 2000) of the Italian pig gene bank.

Breed	Number of		Doses[1]
	Boars	Sires of boars (average kinship among boars)	
Casertana	11	5 (0.19)	800
Cinta Senese	12	8 (0.24)	1000
Mora Romagnola	5	3	400
Nera Siciliana	19	19	1600
Total	47		3800

[1]Dose defined in table 2.

7. The situation of pig cryopreservation in Spain

In Spain the conservation of domestic animal germplasm is regulated by the Ministry of Agriculture on two levels, co-ordination and development. Recently, the Spanish Committee for Animal Reproduction and Gene Banks has been created to co-ordinate the activities of the gene banks, regional and national. As to development, a National Gene Bank has been created in the Centre of Animal Selection and Reproduction of Colmenar Viejo (Madrid). At the same time, the autonomous regions must develop their own regional gene banks.

Work has begun on the pig supported by the EU project RESGEN12 and other national funds coming from the Ministry of Agriculture and research grants. Four different areas of work can be mentioned.

7.1. Infrastructure

We have developed two specific stations for boar training and semen collection together with their respective laboratories, completely equipped for semen freezing and cryoconservation. These stations are organised in 12 stables per variety or breed. A total of 24 boars are maintained simultaneously in the station. These animals are at two different stages: when half of the animals are under collection, the others are under training. When a sufficient number of doses per animal is reached (at least 60-80 by boar), the set is completed and the animals are replaced by a new group of six young animals (six month old) and the animals under training go to collection. We have established a continuous chain to optimise the human and material resources available.

7.2. Technical development

In this area, the traditional technique for semen freezing employed in our laboratories (Westendorf *et al.*, 1975) has been replaced by a new one developed by Thilmant (1997). We have developed a comparative study of the two techniques, using a total number of 70 ejaculates processed with the Thilmant method and another 149 processed with the Westendorf method, and using seven boars (5 *Chato Murciano*, 1 *Negro Iberico* and 1 commercial hybrid).

Our results on subjective parameters (motility and percentage alive) and objective parameters such as vital staining and normal acrosome ring have shown that the Thilmant method improved the Westendorf method by 12% in vital staining and 26% in normal acrosome ring.

Moreover we have developed artificial inseminations using these frozen doses. On a total of 40 sows from four different herds inseminated with doses from the Thilmant method, a mean pregnancy rate around 70% was obtained, reaching 83.3% in some herds. Also, the observed prolificacy of these females was near the values obtained with natural insemination (Poto *et al.*, 2000, in press).

7.3. Training of researchers

The use of the Thilmant method has been recommended to all Spanish laboratories involved in pig semen cryoconservation. To-day this technique, first implemented in the Centre of Agricultural Research and Development (CIDA) in Murcia, is also in use in the University of Cordoba, the University of Lugo and the Centre of Animal Reproduction and Selection (CENSYRA) in Badajoz. Researchers in those laboratories have been trained in the use of the Thilmant method by one of us (A. Poto).

7.4. Gene bank

The freezing operations began in 1997, on 5 boars *Chato Murciano* (CM) and one *Negro Iberico* (NI). The aggressive character of the Iberian boars appeared to be a major obstacle to on-farm collections, and subsequent collections were carried out in the specific stations described above. The present situation of the pig gene bank is presented in Table 7, which shows about 6000 doses stored from 46 boars belonging to 6 different breeds. The doses presently stored in two places, Cordoba and Murcia, will be duplicated in the national gene bank in preparation (see chapter 1.5).

Table 7. Present state (end of 2000) of the Spanish pig gene bank.

Breed	Number of		
	Boars	Sires of boars[1]	Doses[2]
Chato Murciano	16	6	2400
Manchado de Jabugo	5	5	650
Negro Canario	6	6	550
Negro Iberico	5	5	950
Retinto	6	6	900
Torbiscal (Iberian variety)	8	8	550
Total	46	36	6000

[1]Pedigrees not registered except for *Chato Murciano*.
[2]Dose defined in table 2.

8. Discussion and conclusions

It is to-day recognised that the conservation of animal genetic resources has to rely on maintaining local breeds *in situ*, within their specific production systems, *ex situ* conservation appearing as a useful complement. It is also often emphasised that local breeds can only be maintained alive when sufficient economic benefits can be derived from their exploitation. In such a context, cryopreservation has a specific role to play, since there is generally no profit to be expected in the short-medium term. In addition, as shown in Table 2, gene banks are costly to set up. They require an initial investment which needs to be supported outside the routine management of the breed. It should also be reminded that "conservation is a gamble, with a high probability of no pay-off" (Smith, 1984). Storing germplasm may be viewed as a way of preserving a patrimony and taking an insurance against risks of genetic erosion in a more or less distant future. On the other hand, gene banks are also useful tools to support *in situ* conservation, as stressed by Meuwissen (1999), and other achievable objectives have been suggested by FAO-UNEP (1998b). However, it should be stressed that such uses of gene banks are outside the strict domain of long-term conservation, and they need defining specific rules of operation, particularly regarding the number of doses to be stored and their renewal.

Though private initiatives in cryoconservation should be encouraged whenever they appear (*e.g.* in Italy, as mentioned in section 6 of this chapter), a national organisation seems to be necessary. As we have seen, rather precise guidelines have to be followed, in terms of sampling, amount stored and security requirements. The further use and exploitation of the gene banks created also need a careful planning. A legal framework for access to the material stored is needed, given the anticipated lifetime of gene banks and the risk that breeds become extinct and breeders associations no longer exist after the samples were obtained (FAO-UNEP, 1998b). As suggested by FAO, it is therefore advisable that the ownership of the material stored reside with the country of origin, in accordance with the Convention on Biological Diversity. A step in that direction has been made in France with the creation in 1999 of a *Cryobanque Nationale* for all farm animal species. The legal entity so created, which covers the material collected in pigs before and during the RESGEN12 project, has the responsibility of managing the material stored and defining the rules of access. A similar approach is also taken in Spain, as we have seen in section 7.

Table 8. Present state (end of 2000) of the French, German, Italian and Spanish pig gene banks.

Country	Breeds	Number of		Sites of storage
		Boars	Doses[1]	
France	5	135	7 163	2
Germany	2	50	8 588	1[2]
Italy	4	47	3 800	1[2]
Spain	6	46	6 000	2[3]
Total	17	278	25 551	11

[1]Dose defined in the respective country tables 3 4 5 6 7.
[2]Two additional sites in preparation.
[3]One national site in preparation.

To sum up, owing to the support of the RESGEN12 project over the period 1996-2000, four European countries, representing a major part of EU pig production, have now at their disposal a collection of about 25 000 AI doses, representing nearly 280 boars belonging to 17 different local breeds, as shown in Table 8. There is no doubt that the experience so gained will be of some benefit for the management and conservation of pig genetic resources over the whole European continent.

CONCLUSION

In this last part of the book we shall summarise the main results presented in the previous sections and draw some general conclusions. The overall objective of the RESGEN12 project was to establish the bases of a gene bank for the conservation of European genetic resources of pigs, relying in particular on storage of frozen semen from local breeds exposed to serious risks of genetic erosion, if not complete extinction. More specifically, the project intended (1) to characterise a number of local breeds in 4 EU countries and 2 neighbouring Central European countries, (2) to collect data on performances/qualification of each breed, (3) to evaluate the genetic variability within and between breeds, using genetic markers, and (4) to collect germplasm and to apply adequate cryopreservation programmes.

As we have seen, the book is divided up into 4 sections corresponding to the 4 specific objectives just mentioned.

The section on *primary characterisation* offers an overview of the local breeds existing in the 4 countries participating, as well as of their management. General information and so-called "passport data" have been collected on local breeds existing in each country. Pedigree records available have also been analysed. Twenty-three breeds were initially included in the project (*i.e.* FR:6 - DE:8 - IT:5 - ES:4). Some of these, however, had to be discarded, and, inversely, 3 additional native breeds from Spain were added. Overall, 24 breeds were covered, namely 6 French, 4 German, 1 Czech, 1 Polish, 5 Italian and 7 Spanish. Their primary characterisation has been achieved and the relevant information is compiled in various national, regional or global databases, all available on the Internet.

The section on *performances* contains additional information on reproduction and production performances, as well as any specific qualification of the breeds considered. On-farm or experimental station performance records were collected and analysed within each country. They generally confirmed the lower growth and carcass performances of local breeds, however usually compensated by higher meat quality. Special attention was also given to crossbreeding systems including local breeds, as exemplified by the German experiments showing the economic competitiveness of such systems. Possible interactions with environment and specific farming systems were analysed (*e.g.* extensive *vs.* intensive systems in France and Italy). It was stressed that specific farming systems may significantly contribute to breeds' survival. In such a context, the Iberian pig in Southern Spain offers a good example of animal and environment integration, for a product of world reputation, the Iberian acorn ham.

The section on *genetic distances* presents an evaluation of within and between-breed genetic variability, based on blood groups (13 systems), biochemical polymorphisms (11 systems) and DNA simple sequence repeat (13 microsatellite loci), on a subset of 19 breeds (5 FR, 3 DE, 1 CZ, 1 PL, 5 IT and 4 ES). The genetic distances among those 19 breeds were used to derive a diversity function allowing to estimate the contribution of each individual breed, or any breed combination, to the overall diversity. The analysis showed highly unequal breed contributions to the overall diversity. This section should thus provide useful information for establishing conservation priorities both within and among the participating countries.

The last section on *semen banks* describes the *ex situ* conservation programmes operated in each country and presents the status of the collected germplasm at the end of the project. Overall, the stores amount to about 25 000 doses of semen for artificial insemination, collected from 278 boars belonging to 17 breeds. This section also includes a review of the state of the art in cryopreservation techniques and offers practical recommendations for establishing gene banks from local breeds in danger of extinction.

The experience acquired in the project allows to draw some conclusions and to assess its respective tasks' feasibility. It appears that, apart from the genetic distancing task, which was considerably delayed for various reasons, the other 3 tasks did progress quite satisfactorily. From the exchanges having occurred between the partners during the project, it is also quite clear that the situation of the pig genetic resources, and the attention paid to their evaluation and conservation, may vary considerably from one country to another. This EU-supported co-operation thus appears to have fulfilled the following two useful roles: either to provide a stimulus for additional support by the country's own financial resources (*e.g.* Italy and Spain), or to bring a substantial complementary support to the national policies already implemented (e.g. France and Germany).

The project scope has been enhanced by a demonstration project on pig biodiversity (PIGBIODIV: BIO4-CT98-0188) run in parallel. In PIGBIODIV, the RESGEN12 participants 3 (DE), 4 (IT) and 5 (ES) operated as subcontractors to participant 1 (FR), and as such they realised the necessary breeds sampling and DNA extraction in their respective countries. PIGBIODIV allowed carrying to completion the analysis of a pilot diversity study funded by EC in 1994-96 within the Pig Gene Mapping Project (PiGMaP). The paper published (Laval *et al.,* 2000) gives an evaluation of genetic distances between 11 European breeds, including wild pigs, major commercial breeds and local breeds, among which 5 breeds (4 FR, 1 DE) included in this project. It was shown, in particular, that the 4 French local breeds, though representing less than 0.1 % of the total French sow population, accounted for about half of the total genetic diversity of the 11 breeds included in the pilot study. This is an indication of the potential impact of preserving local endangered breeds on the maintenance of a species biodiversity. A much larger sample of European breeds (including commercial lines) and countries was covered in the PIGBIODIV demonstration project. The data collected are currently being analysed and should thus extend and complement the diversity analysis carried on in this project.

The work carried out has made clear the need to develop sound conservation programmes that will integrate *ex situ* strategies, such as semen conservation, with the maintenance of local endangered breeds within economically sustainable production systems. As said in conclusion of the foreword to this book, it is hoped that those results will help in the management and conservation of pig genetic resources over the whole European continent and in other countries of the world as well. The book is also likely to stimulate further work for extending our knowledge of the pig and other farm animal species genetic diversity.

REFERENCES

A.O.A.C., 1980. Official methods of Analysis (13th Ed.). Association of Official Analytical Chemist, Washington D.C.

Abeydeera L.R., Johonson L.A., Welch G.R., Wang W.H., Boquest A.C., Canrley T.C., Rieke A., Day B.N., 1998. Birth of piglets preselected for gender following *in vitro* fertilization of *in vitro* matured pig oocytes by X and Y chromosome bearing spermatozoa sorted by high speed flow cytometry. Ther., 50, 981-988.

Archibald A., 1997. The pig gene mapping project (PiGMaP). In Hoeveler A. Cresti M. (Eds). Biotechnology (1992-1994). Final Report. Official Publication of the European Immunities, Luxembourg, vol. 2, 193-207.

Archibald A., Haley C.S., Brown J., Couperwhite S., McQueen H.A., 1995. The PiGMaP consortium linkage map of the pig (*Sus scrofa*). Mamm. Genome, 6, 157-175.

Baguisi A., Overström E.W., 2000. Induced enucleation in nuclear transfer procedures to produce cloned animals. Ther., 53, 209.

Barba C., 1999. Caracterización productiva de las variedades del cerdo Ibérico como base para su conservación. PhD Thesis Universidad de Córdoba.

Barba C., Forero J., M. Cumbreras M.,. Sanz M.,. Suárez M.V., Delgado. J.V., 1999. Análisis de la situación genética de la raza Manchado de Jabugo. III Congreso de la SERGA y I Ibérico de conservación de RGA. Lugo, España.

Barker J.S.F., 2001. Conservation and management of genetic diversity: a domestic animal perspective. Can. J. For. Res., 31, 588-595.

Barker J.S.F., Hill W.G., Bradley D., Nei M., Fries R., Wayne R.K., 1993. An integrated global programme to establish the genetic relationships among the breeds of each domestic animal species. FAO, Rome. Reprinted as FAO, 1998. Secondary Guidelines for Development of National Farm Animal Genetic Resources Management Plans. Measurement of Domestic Animal Diversity (MoDAD): Original Working Group Report. FAO, Rome.

Bejerhom C., Barton-Gade P., 1986. Effect of intramuscular fat level on eating quality of pig meat. Proceedings of the 32nd European meeting of meat research workers, Gent, Belgium, 389-391.

Berthelot F., Martinat-Botté F., Locatelli A., Terqui M., 2000. Piglets born after vitrification of embryos using the Open Pulled Straw method. Cryobiol., 41, 116-124.

Betthauser J., Forsberg E., Augenstein M., Childs L., Eilertsen K., Enos J., Forsythe T., Jurgella G., Koppang R., Lesmeister T., Mallon K., Mell G., Misica P., Pace M., Pfister-Genskow M., Strelchenko N., Voelker G., Watt S., Thompson S., Bishop M. 2000. Production of cloned pigs from *in vitro* systems. Nat. Biotech., 18, 1055-1059.

Blecher S.R., Howie, Detmar J., Blahunt L.M., 1999. A new approach to immunological sexing of sperm. Ther., 52, 1309-1321.

Brem G., Graf F., Kräusslich H., 1984. Genetic and economic differences among methods of gene conservation in Livest. Prod. Sci., 11,65-68.

Bühler R., 1987. Das Schwäbisch-Hällische Schwein. Alte Rasse mit aktuellen Eigenschaften. Schweinezucht u. Schweinemast 35, 152-155.

Bühler R., 1997. Das Schwäbisch-Hällische Landschwein - älteste und traditionsreichste Schweinerasse Deutschlands. In: Gefährdete Schweinerassen, GEH/Hörning, NZH-Verlag Wetzlar. 21-26.

Bussière J.F., Bertaud G., Guillouet P., 2000. Conservation de la semence congelée de verrat. Résultats *in vitro* et après insémination. Journées Rech. Porcine en France, 32, 429-432.

Campbell K.H.S., Mc Whir J., Ritchie W.A.R., Wilmut I., 1996. Sheep cloned by nuclear transfer from a cultured cell line. Nat., 380, 64-66.

Campodoni G., Franci O., Acciaioli A., 1999. In vita performances and carcass traits of Large White x Cinta Senese pigs reared outdoor and indoor. Proceedings A.S.P.A. XIII Meeting, 555-557.

Cañon J., Alexandrino P., Bessa I., Carleos C., Carretero Y., Dunner S., Ferran N., Garcia D., Jordana J., Laloë D., Pereira A., Sanchez A., Moazami-Goudarzi K., 2001. Genetic diversity measures of local European beef cattle breeds for conservation purposes. Genet. Sel. Evol., 33, 311-322.

Canope I., Raynaud Y., 1980. Etude comparative des performances de reproduction des truies de races Créole et Large White en Guadeloupe. Ann. Génét. Sél. Anim., 12, 267.

Canope I., Raynaud Y., 1981. Comparative study of the reproduction and the fattening performance of Creole and Large White pigs in Guadeloupe. 32nd Annual Meeting of EAAP. Zagreb, 31/08-03/09, 1-5.

Chainetr W., 2001. Systematische Gebrauchskreuzung als Möglichkeit der Erhaltung vom Aussterben bedrohter Landrassen. Dissertation Univ. Göttingen.

Cheng P.L., 1984. Livestock Breeds of China. FAO Animal Production and Health Paper n° 46, Rome.

Cibelli J.B., Stice S.L., Golueke P.J., Kane J.J., Jerry J., Blackwell C., Ponce de Leon A., Robl J.M., 1998. Cloned transgenic calves produced from non-quiescent fetal fibroblasts. Sci., 280, 1256-1258.

Clemens R., Meyer J.-N., 1996. Elektrophoretische Methoden zur Identifizierung von biochemischen Polymorphismen. Laborhandbuch.

Colatruglio P., Girolami A., Grasso F., Napolitano F., Palazzo M., Zullo A., Matassino D., 1996. Confronto fra suini "Casertana" e suoi derivati. I. Alcuni rilievi alla mattazione. Prod. Anim., IX(III), suppl., 119-123.

Colman A., 2000. Somatic cell Nuclear Transfer in mammals: progress and applications. Cloning, 1, 185-200.

Comberg G., 1978. Schweinezucht. 8th Ed., Verlag E. Ulmer, Stuttgart.

Córdova A., Ducolomb Y., Jiménez I., Casas E., Bonilla E., Betancourt M., 1997. *In vitro* fertilizing capacity of frozen-thawed boar semen. Ther., 47, 1309-1317.

Coutron-Gambotti C., Gandemer G., Casabianca F., 1998. Effects of substituting a concentrate diet for chestnuts on the lipid traits of muscle and adipose tissues in Corsican and Corsican x Large White pigs reared in a sylvo-pastoral system in Corsica. Meat Sci., 50, 163-174.

Darin-Bennet A., White I.G., 1977. Influences of cholesterol content of mammalian spermatozoa on susceptibility to cold-shock. Cryobiology, 14, 466-470.

Delatte J.J., Le Guyadec P., Le Duot P., Duclos J.M., 1991. Croissance et reproduction des porcs rustiques d'origine française selon le milieu d'élevage en Haiti. Journées Rech., Porcine en France, 23, 381-388.

Delgado J.V., Barba C., Dieguez E., Cañuelo P., Herrera M., Rodero A., 1998. "Caracterización exteriorista de las variedades del cerdo Ibérico basada en caracteres cualitativos". En: II Congreso Nacional de la Sociedad Española para los Recursos Genéticos Animales (SERGA). Mallorca.

Delgado J.V., Barba C., Poto A., Sánchez L., Calero R., Fresno M.R. 2000a. "Conservation programme of the Spanish pig genetic resources". Options Méditerranéennes, Ciheam, ICAM-UE. 41, 53-56.

Delgado J.V., Barba C., Dieguez E., Cañuelo P., Herrera M., Rodero A., 2000b. "Morphological characterization of the Iberian pig branch based on quantitative traits". Options Méditerranéennes, Ciheam, ICAM-UE. 41, 63-66.

Didion B.A., Pomp D., Martin M.J., Homanics G.E., Markert C.L., 1990. Observations on the cooling and cryopreservation of pig oocytes at the germinal vesicle stage. J. Anim. Sci., 68, 2803-2810.

Dinklage H., Gruhn R.,1969. Blutgruppen-and Serumproteinpolymorphisms bei verchiedenen in Deutschland vorhandenen Schweinerassen. Z. Tierzücht. Züchtbiol., 86, 136-146.

Dobrinsky J.R., 1997. Cryopreservation of pig embryos. J. Reprod Fertil Suppl., 52, 301-312.

Dobrinsky J.R., Johnson L.A., 1994. Cryopreservation of porcine embryos by vitrification: a study of *in vitro* development. Ther., 42, 25-35.

Dobrinsky J.R., Pursel V.G., Long C.R., Johnson L.A., 2000. Birth of piglets after transfer of embryos cryopreserved by cytoskeletal stabilization and vitrification. Biol. Rep., 62, 564-570.

Dominko T., Ramalho-Santos J., Chan A., Moreno R.D., 1999. Optimization strategies for production of mammalian embryos by nuclear transfer. Cloning, 1, 143-152.

Dondi G., 1924. La razza suina Cinta. Rivista di Zootecnia, 1, 237-245.

Dutertre J.B., 1667-1671. Histoire des Antilles, 3 vol. 4 tomes. Nouvelle réédition 1958, Société d'histoire de la Martinique C.E.P. Fort de France.

Ehlich M., 1997. Das Deutsche Sattelschwein. In: Gefährdete Schweinerassen, GEH/Hörning, NZH-Verlag Wetzlar. 27-32.

Enfält A.C., Lundström K., Hansson I., Lundeheim N., Nyström P.E., 1997. Effect of Outdoor rearing and sire breed (Duroc or Yorkshire) on carcass composition and sensory and technological meat quality. Meat Sci., 45, 1-15.

Epstein H., 1969. Domestic Animals of China. CAB, England.

Epstein H., 1971. The Origin of the Domestic Animals of Africa. Vol. 2. Africana Publishing Corporation, New York.

Epstein H., Bichard M., 1984. Pig. In: Evolution of Domesticated Animals (I.L. Mason ed.), Longman, 145-162.

Eriksson B.M., Rodriguez-Martinez H., 1999. Export of frozen boar semen in a new flat package. Proceedings of IV International Conference on Boar Semen Preservation, Belstville, Maryland USA. P26.

Eriksson B.M., Rodriguez-Martinez H., 2000. Deep-freezing of boar semen in plastic film 'cochettes'. Zentralbl Veterinarmed A., 47, 89-97.

Evans M.J., Gurer C., Loike J.D., Wilmut I., Schnieke E., Schon E.A., 1999. Mitochondrial DNA genotypes in nuclear transfer-derived cloned sheep. Nat. Gen., 23, 90-93.

Falconer D.S., 1989. Introduction to Quantitative Genetics. Longman Scientific & Technical, Essex, England.

FAO 1998a. Report of Workshop New developments in biotechnology and their implications for the conservation of farm animal genetic resources. Reversible DNA quiescence and somatic cloning. FAO, Rome, Italy, 26-28 November 1997.

FAO-UNEP, 1998b. Secondary guidelines for development of national farm animal genetic resources management plans. Management of small populations at risk. FAO, Rome, 229 pp.

Feroci S., 1979. Salvare le razze italiane. Rivista di Suinicoltura, 10,13-19.

Forero J., 1999. "Estudio comparativo de cinco estirpes de cerdo Ibérico". Excma. Diputación Provincial de Huelva. 230 pp.

Forero J., Cumbreras M., Venegas M., Ferrer N., Barba C., Delgado J.V., 1999. Contribución a la caracterización productiva del Manchado de Jabugo en el periodo predestete: resultados preliminares. In: III Congreso de la SERGA y I Ibérico de conservación de RGA. Lugo, España.

Foulley J.L., Hill W.G., 1999. On the precision of estimation of genetic distance. Genet. Sel. Evol., 31, 457-464.

Franci O., Baldini P., Bozzi R., Bellatti M., Pugliese C., Acciaioli A., Geri G., 1997. Confronto fra progenie di verri Large White, Landrace Italiana, Landrace Belga, Duroc, Cinta Senese e scrofe Large White a 130 e 160 kg di peso vivo. 5. Caratteristiche tecnologiche e sensoriali del prosciutto toscano. Zoot. Nutr. Anim, 23, 67-79.

Franci O., Bozzi R., Pugliese C., Poli B.M., Parisi G., Balo' F., Geri G.. 1995. Confronto fra progenie di verri Large White, Landrace Italiana, Landrace Belga, Duroc, Cinta Senese e scrofe Large White a 130 e 160 kg di peso vivo. 3. Caratteristiche fisico-chimiche del magro e del grasso della coscia. Zoot. Nutr. Anim., 21, 237-247.

Franci O., Poli B.M., Pugliese C., Bozzi R., Parisi G., Balo' F., Geri G., 1996. Confronto fra progenie di verri Large White, Landrace Italiana, Landrace Belga, Duroc, Cinta Senese e scrofe Large White a 130 e 160 kg di peso vivo. 4. Caratteristiche fisico-chimiche del prosciutto toscano. Zoot. Nutr. Anim., 22, 149-158.

Franci O., Pugliese C., Acciaioli A., Campodoni G., Bozzi R., Gandini G. 2000. Caratteristiche chimico-fisiche della carne di suini Cinta Senese, Large White e relativi incroci in condizioni di allevamento intensivo. In "Tradition et Innovation dans la production porcine méditerranéenne". Alfonso de Almeida et Tirapicos Nunes (eds), Options Méditerranéennes A, 41, 201-204.

Franci O., Pugliese C., Acciaioli A., Poli B.M., Geri G., 1994a. Confronto fra progenie di verri Large White, Landrace Italiana, Landrace Belga, Duroc, Cinta Senese e scrofe Large White a 130 e 160 kg di peso vivo. 1. Rilievi in vita e alla macellazione. Zoot. Nutr. Anim., 20, 129-142.

Franci O., Pugliese C., Bozzi R., Parisi G., Acciaioli A., Geri G., 1994b. Confronto fra progenie di verri Large White, Landrace Italiana, Landrace Belga, Duroc, Cinta Senese e scrofe Large White a 130 e 160 kg di peso vivo. 2. Composizione della carcassa e caratteristiche del coscio. Zoot. Nutr. Anim., 20, 177-186.

Fredeen H.T., 1984. Selection limits: have they been reached with pigs? Can. J. Anim. Sci., 64, 223-234.

Galli C., Duchi R., Moor R.M., Lazzari G., 1999. Mammalian leukocytes contain all the genetic information necessary for the development of a new individual. Cloning, 1, 161-170.

Gandini G., Oldenbroek J.K., 1999. Choosing the conservation strategy. In "Genebanks and the conservation of farm animal genetic resources". J.K. Oldenbroek, (eds.) 11-31, ID-DLO, Lelystad, The Netherlands.

Gandini G., Orlandini P., Franci O., Campodoni G., 2000. Hypothesis for decreasing inbreeding in the Cinta Senese pig. Options Méditerranéennes, A - 41, 35-37.

GEH/Hörning B., 1997. Gefährdete Schweinerassen und Alternative Züchtung. GEH und NZH-Verlag, Wetzlar (ISBN 3-92687-25-X).

Gibson J.P., Freeman A.E., Boettcher P.J. 1997. Cytoplasmic and mitochondrial inheritance of economic traits in cattle. Livest. Prod. Sci., 47, 115-124.

Girolami A., Colatruglio P., D'Agostino N., Grasso F., Napolitano F., Zullo A., Matassino D., 1996. Confronto fra suini "Casertana" e suoi derivati. III. Alcuni rilievi allo spolpo della carcassa. Prod. Anim., IX(III), suppl., 131-134.

Giuliani R., 1940. Le razze suine allevate in Italia. Rivista di Zootecnia, 11-12, 412-428.

Glodek P., 1963. Die Züchtung eines Deutschen Fleischschweines unter dem Einfluss holländischer Veredelter Landschweine. Züchtungskunde 35, 54-63.

Glodek P., 1991. Evaluation and utilization of pig breeds. In: Genetic Resources of Pig, Sheep and Goats (K. Maijala ed.), 65-93, Elsevier.

Glodek P., 2000. Theorie und Praxis der Konservierung tiergenetischer Ressourcen am Beispiel zweier alter deutscher Schweinerassen (pp. 31-41). In: Festsymposium D.L. Simon 11.8.2000. Hrsg. O. Distl, Hieronymus, München.

Glodek P., Brandt H., Meyer J.N., Götz K.U., 1990. Is the Angeln Saddleback pig a genetic resource for future animal production? World. Rev. Anim. Prod. XXV (1),13-16.

Glodek P., Meyer J.N., Brandt H., Pfeiffer H., 1993. Die genetische Distanz zwischen ost- und west-deutschen Schweinerassen. 1. Mitteilung: Die Eigenständigkeit und der Heterozygotiegrad der Rassen. Archiv f. Tierz. 36, 621-630.

Goumy S., 1999. Comparaison de quatre races locales porcines pour les performances de croissance, carcasse et qualité de la viande. Mémoire de recherche, E.S.I.T.PA., 65 pp.

Grasso F., Cappuccio A., Colatruglio P., Girolami A., Napolitano F., Zullo A., Matassino D., 1996. Confronto fra suini "Casertana" e suoi derivati. II. Alcuni rilievi alla sezionatura della carcassa. Prod. Anim., IX(III), suppl., 125-129.

Grau R., Hamm R. 1952. Eine einfache Methode zur Bestimmung der Wasserbindung im Fleich. Fleischwirtschaft, 4, 295-297.

Gregorius H.-R., 1974. Genetischer Abstand zwischen Populationen. Silvae Genetica, 23, 1-3.

Greider C.W., 1996. Telomere length regulation. Ann. Rev. Bioch., 65, 337-365.

Guerrero L., Gou P., Arnau J., 1999. The influence of meat pH on mechanical and sensory textural properties of dry-cured ham. Meat Sci., 52, 267-273.

Haring, F., 1961. In: Handbuch der Tierzüchtung, Bd. 3(2) Rassenkunde. Hammond, Johansson, Haring. Verlag P. Parey, Hamburg-Berlin.

Hill W.G., 1993. Variation in genetic composition in backcrossing programs. J. Hered., 84, 212-213.

I.T.P., 1999. Les Races Porcines Françaises. Techni-Porc, 22 (4), dépliant détachable.

IGR/ZADI, Oetmann I., 2000. Genetische Resourcen für Ernährung, Landwirtschaft und Forsten. Angew. Wiss. Heft 487; Schriftenreihe BML.

Jaume J., Alfonso L., Pérez-Enciso M., 1997. Estado actual y perspectivas de conservación del cerdo Negro Mallorquín. In: I Congreso de la Sociedad Española de Genética. Valencia.

Jaume J., Cifre J., Puigserver G., 1999. Parámetros reproductivos del cerdo negro mallorquín. In: III Congreso de la SERGA y I Ibérico de conservación de RGA. Lugo, España.

Johnson L.A., Guthrie H.D., Dobrinsky J.R., Welch G.R. 2000a. Low dose artificial insemination of swine with sperm sorted for sex using intrauterine technique in sows. Proceedings of the 14th ICAR, Stockholm, July 2000. 244.

Johnson L.A., Guthrie H.D., Fiser P., Maxwell W.M.C., Welch G.R., Garrett W.M. 2000b. Cryopreservation of flow cytometrically sorted boar sperm: effects on *in vivo* embryo development. J. Anim, 78 (Suppl. 1), Abstr. (in press).

Johnson L.A., Welch G.R. 1999. Sex preselection: high-speed flow cytometric sorting of X and Y sperm for maximum efficiency. Ther., 52,1323-1341.

Jonsson P., 1991. Civilization and domestication of pigs. In: Genetic Resources of Pig, Sheep and Goats (K. Maijala ed.), 11-50, Elsevier.

Kawarasaki T., Matsumoto K, Murofushi J., Chikyu M., Itagaki Y and Horiuchi A. 2000. Sexing of porcine embryo by in situ hybridization using chromosome Y- and 1-specific DNA probes. Ther., 53, 1501-1509.

King J.W.B., 1991. Pig breeds of the world: their distribution and adaptation. In: Genetic Resources of Pig, Sheep and Goats (K. Maijala ed.), 51-63, Elsevier.

King J.W.B., 1992. Genetic improvement and conservation of Taihu pig breeds in Jiangsu province (draft report).

King W. 1999. Telomeres and telomerase activity in bovine oocytes, embryos and fetuses. Ther., 49, 182.

Kober H., 1992. Das Schwäbisch-Hällische Schwein. Bestandsaufnahme einer gefährdeten Nutztierrasse. Diss. TiHo Hannover.

Kolbe T., Holtz W. 1999. Intracytoplasmatic injection (ICSI) of *in vivo* or *in vitro* matured oocytes with fresh ejaculated or frozen thawed epididymal spermatozoa and additional calcium-ionophore activation in the pig. Ther., 52, 671-682.

Kubota C., Yamakuchi H., Todoroki J., Mizoshita K., Tabara N., Barber M., Yang X. 2000. Six cloned calves produced from adult fibroblasts cells after long-term culture. Proc. Nat. Acad. Sci. USA, 97), 990-995.

Kubota C., Yang X., Dinnyes A., Todoroki J., Yamakuchi H., Mizoshita K., Inohae S., Tabara N. 1998. *In vitro* and *in vivo* survival of frozen-thawed bovine oocytes after IVF, nuclear transfer, and partenogenetic activation. Mol. Rep. Dev., 51, 281-286.

Labat C., 1722. Nouveau voyage aux Isles de l'Amérique. Cavelier, Paris 6 vol. (nombreuses rééditions).

Labroue F., Goumy S., Gruand J., Mourot J., Neelz V., Legault C., 2000a. Comparaison au Large White de quatre races locales porcines françaises pour les performances de croissance, de carcasse et de qualité de la viande. Journées Rech. Porcine en France, 32, 403-411.

Labroue F., Guillouet P., Marsac H., Boisseau C., Luquet M., Arrayet J., Martinat-Botté F., Terqui M., 2000b. Etude des performances de reproduction de 5 races locales porcines françaises. Journées Rech. Porcine en France, 32, 413-418.

Labroue F., Luquet M., 1999. Les races locales porcines françaises. Techni-Porc, 22 (1), 17-19.

Larsson K., Einarsson S., Swensson T. 1977. The development of a practicable method for deep freezing of boar spermatozoa. Nord. Vet. Med., 29, 113-118.

Lauvergne J.J., 1982. Genetica en problaciones animales después de la domestication: consecuencias para la conservacion de las razas. 2nd World Congress Genet. Appl. Livest. Prod., 6, 77-87.

Lauvergne J.J., Canope I., 1979. Etude de quelques variants colorés du porc Créole de la Guadeloupe. Ann. Génét. Sél. Anim., 11, 381.

Laval G., Iannucelli N., Legault C., Milan D., Groenen M.A.M., Giuffra E., Andersson L., Nissen P.H., Jorgensen C.B., Beeckman P., Geldermann H., Foulley J.L., Chevalet C., Ollivier L., 2000. Genetic diversity of eleven European pig breeds. Genet. Sel. Evol., 32,: 187-203.

Laval G., San Cristobal-Gaudy M., Chevalet C., 2001. Measuring genetic distances between breeds: use of some distances in various short term evolution models. Genet. Sel. Evol. (submitted).

Legault C., 1978. Particularités zootechniques des porcs élevés en République Populaire de Chine. Bull. Tech. Inf. n° 327: 115-125.

Legault C., Audiot A., Daridan D., Gruand J., Lagant H., Luquet M., Molénat M., Rouzade D., Simon M.N., 1996. Recherche de références sur les possibilités de valoriser les porcs Gascon et Limousin par des produits de qualité. 1 Engraissement, carcasses, coûts de production. Journées Rech. Porcine en France, 28, 115-122.

Legault C., Caritez J.C., 1983. L'expérimentation sur le porc chinois en France. I. Performances de reproduction en race pure et en croisement. Génét. Sél. Evol., 15, 225-240.

Li M.D., Enfield F.D., 1989. A characterization of Chinese breeds of swine using cluster analysis. J. Anim. Breed. Genet., 106, 379-388.

Lo L.L., McLaren D.G., McKeith F.K., Fernando R.L., Novakofski J. 1992. Genetic analyses of growth, real-time ultrasound, carcass, and pork quality traits in Duroc and Landrace pigs: I. Breed effects. J. Anim. Sci., 70, 2373-2386.

Lömker R. and Simon D. L., 1994. Costs of and inbreeding in conservation strategies for endangered breeds of cattle. Proc. 5th World Congr. Genet. Appl. Livestock Prod., 21, 393-396.

López J. L., A. Argüello, J. Capote and N. Darmanin. 1992. Contribution to the study of Black Canary Pig. *Archivos de Zootecnia.* Vol 41 (extra), 531-536.

Macháty Z., Rickords L.F., Prather R.S. 1999. Parthenogenetic activation of porcine oocytes after nuclear transfer. Cloning, 1, 101-109.

Major F., 1968. Untersuchungen über die verwandtschaftlichen Beziehungen zwischen verschiedenen europäischen Landrassepopulationen mit Hilfe von Blutgruppenfaktoren. PhD thesis. Univ. Göttingen.

Mannen H., Kojima T., Oyama K., Mukai F., Ishida T., Tsuji S. 1998. Effect of mitochondrial DNA variation on carcass traits of Japaneese Black cattle. J. Anim. Sci., 76, 36-41.

Mariante A., 1990. Programmes for live animal preservation for Latin America. FAO Animal Production and Health paper n° 80, 119-126.

Marsac H., Luquet M., Labroue F., 1999. Premier bilan annuel des performances de reproduction des 5 races locales porcines françaises. Techni-Porc, 22 (5), 31-39.

Martínez A.M, de la Haba M., Zamorano M.J., Rodero A., Vega-Pla J.L., 1998 Characterization of Iberian pig with 25 microsatellites based on multiplex PCR. Animal Genetics 29 (Suppl. 1), 10-23.

Martínez A.M., Rodero A., Vega-Pla J.L. 2000a. Estudio con microsatélites de las principales variedades de ganado Porcino del tronco Ibérico. Arch Zootec., 49, 45-52.

Martínez A.M., Delgado J.V., Rodero A., Vega-Pla J.L.2000b. Genetic structure of the Iberian pig breed using microsatellites. Animal Genetics, 31, 295-301.

Martínez A.M., Peinado B., Barba C., Delgado J.V., Vega-Pla J.L. 2000c. Genetic analysis of the Chato Murciano pig and its relationships with the Iberian pig using microsatellites. In: 27th International Society of Animal Genetics, ISAG. Minneapolis, USA.

Mascheroni E., 1927. Zootecnia Speciale, Unione Tipografico-Editrice Torinese, Torino.

Mason J.L. 1988. A World Dictionary of Livestock Breeds Types and Varieties. CAB International, 348 pp.

Mata C., Pardo J., Barba C., Rodero A., Delgado J.V., Molina A., Dieguez E., Cañuelo P., 1998. Estudio morfométrico en las variedades negras del cerdo ibérico. Arch. Zootec., 47, 178-179.

Mathes Maite, 1996. Sattelschweine in Deutschland - Genanteile, Verwandtschaft, Inzucht. Diss. TiHo Hannover.

Mayoral A.I., Dorado M., Guillén M.T., Robina A., Vivo J.M., Vázquez C., Ruiz J., 1999. Development of meat and carcass quality characteristics in Iberian pigs reared outdoors. Meat Sci., 52, 315-324.

McEvoy T.G., Coull G.D., Broadbent P.J., Hutchinson J.S.M. and Speake B.K. 2000. Fatty acid composition of lipids in immature cattle, pig and sheep oocytes with intact zona pellucida. J.Reprod. Fertil., 118, 163-170.

Meuwissen T.H.E. 1999. Operation of conservation schemes. In "Genebanks and the conservation of farm animal genetic resources". J.K. Oldenbroek (ed.), 91-112. ID-DLO Institute for Animal Science and Health, Lelystad, The Netherlands.

Molénat M., Legault C. and Sellier P., 1992. Bases génétiques objectives de la production d'une viande de porc de haute qualité dans le Sud de la France. 2ème Colloque porc méditerranéen Badajoz 25-27 mars.

Molénat M., Legault C., 1986. Le porc dans les pays en voie de développement. Quelques pistes d'amélioration. Bull. tech. Inf. n° 406, 39-53.

Molénat M., Tran The Thong, 1991. Génétique et Elevage du Porc au Vietnam. Institut d'Elevage et de Médecine Vétérinaire des Pays Tropicaux, Maisons-Alfort, France.

Nagashima H., Ashman R.J., Nottle M.B. 1997. Nuclear transfer of porcine embryos using cryopreserved delipated blastomeres as donor nuclei. Mol. Reprod. Dev., 48, 339-343.

Nei M., 1972. Genetic distances between populations. Amer. Nat., 106, 283-292.

Nei M., 1987. Molecular Evolutionary Genetics. Columbia University Press, New York.

Ogura A., Inoue K., Ogonuki N., Noguchi A., Takano K., Nagano R., Suzuki O., Lee J., Ishino F., Matsuda J. 2000a. Production of male cloned mice from fresh, cultured, and cryopreserved immature Sertoli Cells. Biol. Rep., 62, 1579-1584.

Ogura A., Inoue K., Takano K., Wakayama T., Yanagimachi R. 2000b. Production of mice after nuclear transfer by electrofusion using tail tip cells. Mol. Rep. Dev., 57, 55-59.

Ollivier L., 1998. Animal genetic resources in Europe: present situation and future prospects for conservation. The 8th World Conference on Animal Production, Seoul, Korea. Proceedings Symposium Series I, 237-244.

Ollivier L., Bodo I., Simon D.L., 1994. Current developments in the conservation of domestic animal diversity in Europe. 5th World Congr. Genet. Appl. Livestock Prod., 21, 455-461.

Ollivier L., Lagant H., Gruand J., Molénat M., 1991. Progrès génétique des porcs Large White et Landrace français de 1977 à 1987. Journées Rech. Porcine en France, 23, 389-394.

Ollivier L., Lauvergne J.J. 1988. Development and utilization of animal genetic resources. Proc. VI World Conference on Animal Production 27 June 1 July 1988, Helsinki, 85-101.

Ollivier L., Molénat M., 1992. A global review of the genetic resources of pigs. In: The management of global animal genetic resources (J. Hodges ed.). FAO Animal Production and Health paper n° 104, 177-187, FAO, Rome.

Ollivier L., Renard J.P. 1995. The costs of cryopreservation of animal genetic resources. 46th Annual Meeting EAAP – Prague 4-7 September 1995, 7 pp.

Ollivier L., Sellier P., 1983. Pig genetics: a review. Ann. Génét. Sél. Evol., 14, 481-544.

Onishi A., Iwamoto M., Akita T., Mikawa S., Takeda K., Awata T., Hanada H., Perry A.C.F. 2000. Pig cloning by microinjection of fetal fibroblasts nuclei. Sci., 289, 1189-1190.

Panepinto L.M., Phillips R.W., Wheeler L.R., Hill D.H., 1978. The Yucatan miniature pig as a laboratory animal. Laboratory Anim. Sci., 28, 308-313.

Paquignon M., Courot M.1976. Fertlizing capacity of frozen boar spermatozoa. Proc VIIIth Int. Congr. Anim Reprod. and AI, Kracow 1976, 4, 1041-1044.

Paquignon M., Quellier P., Dacheux J.L., 1986. Congélation du sperme de verrat: comparaison de différents dilueurs, techniques de préparation de la semence, mode de conditionnement et température de décongélation. Ann. Zootech., 35, 173-194.

Pardo J., Mata C., Barba C. Rodero A., Delgado J.V., Molina A. Dieguez E. Cañuelo P., 1998. Estudio morfométrico en las variedades rojas del cerdo ibérico. Arch. Zootec., 47, 178-179.

Parks J.E. and Lynch J.V. 1992. Lipid composition and thermotropic phase behaviour of boar, bull, stallion and rooster sperm membranes. Cryobiology, 29, 255-266.

Pathiraja N., Oyedipe E.O., 1990. Indigenous pigs of Nigeria. Bulletin d'Information sur les Ressources Génétiques Animales, n° 7, 67-68, FAO Rome.

Payeras Ll. 1998. El Porc Negre Marllorquí. In: Els animals doméstics de raça autóctona de Mallorca". PRAM, Palma de Mallorca. 160 pp.

Peinado B., Poto A., Marín M., Lobera J.B., 1999. Parámetros productivos del cerdo Chato Murciano (estudio preliminar). En: III Congreso de la Sociedad Española para los Recursos Genéticos Animales(S.E.R.G.A.) y I Congreso Ibérico sobre los Recursos Genéticos Animales. (C.I.R.G.A.), Lugo 1999.

Persidis A. 1999. Xenotransplantation. Nat. Biot., 17, 205-206.

Peura T.T., Lane M.W., Vajta G., Trounson A.O. 1999. Cloning of bovine embryos from vitrified donor blastomeres. J. Rep. Fertil., 116, 95-101.

Peura T.T., Trounson A.O. 1999. Recycling bovine embryos for nuclear transfer. Rep. Fert. Dev., 10, 627-632.

Pfeiffer H., 1988. Schweinezucht, 4. Aufl. Deutscher Landwirtschaftsverlag Berlin.

Polejaeva I.A., Campbell K.H. 2000. New advances in somatic cell nuclear transfer: application in transgenesis. Ther., 53, 117-126.

Polejaeva I.A., Chen S.H., Vaught T.D., Page R.L., Mullins J., Ball Y., Boone J., Walker S., Ayares D.L., Colman A., Campbell K. 2000. Cloned pigs produced by nuclear transfer from adult somatic cells. Nature, 407, 86-90.

Polge C., Salamon S., Wilmut I., 1970. Fertilizing capacity of frozen boar semen following surgical insemination. Vet. Rec., 87, 424-429.

Pollard J.W. and Leibo S.P. 1994. Chilling sensitivity of mammalian embryos. Ther., 41, 101-106.

Popescu C. P., Boscher J., Malynicz G. L.,1989. Chromosome R-banding patterns and NOR homologies in the European wild pig and four breeds of domestic pigs. Ann. Génét., 32, 136-140.

Porter V., 1993. Pigs: a handbook to the breeds of the world, Helm Information Ltd, The Banks East Sussex, 256 pp.

Poto A., Martínez M., Barba C., Peinado B., Lobera J.B. Delgado J.V., 2000. "Ethnozootechnical characterization and analysis of the genetic situation of the Chato Murciano pig breed". Options Méditerranéennes, Ciheam, ICAM-UE. Vol. 41, pp 67-70.

Poto A., Peinado B., Barba C., Delgado J.V., 2000. Congelacion de esperma de verraco de razas autoctonas en peligro de extincion. Influencia de la metodologia en los bancos de germoplasma de pequenas poblaciones.Arch. Zootec., 49, 493-496.

Poulos A., Darin-Bennet A., White I.G. 1973. The phospholipid-bound fatty acids and aldehydes of mammalian spermatozoa. Comp. Biochem. Physiol., 46B, 541-549.

Prather R.S., Sims M.L., First N.L. 1989. Nuclear transplantation in early pig embryos. Biol. Rep., 41, 4141-418.

Prather R.S., Tao T., Macháty Z. 1999. Development of the techniques for nuclear transfer in pigs. Ther., 51, 487-498.

Primo A.T., 1987. Conservation of animal genetic resources: Brazil national programme. FAO Animal Production and Health Paper n° 66, 165-173.

Pursel V.G., Johnson L.A. 1975. Freezing of boar spermatozoa: fertilizing capacity with concentrated semen and a new thawing procedure. J. Anim. Sci., 40, 99-102.

Quittet E., Zert P., 1971. Races porcines en France. La Maison Rustique, Paris, 43 pp.

Ramos A. M., Delgado J.V., Rangel-Figueiredo T., Barba C., Matos J. Cumbreras M., 2000. Genotypic and allelic frequencies of the RYR1 locus in the Manchado de Jabugo pig breed. In: pp 175-178. Quality of meat and fat in pigs as affected by genetics and nutrition. EAAP Publication n° 100. Zurich, Switzerland.

Rath D., Johnson L.A., Dobrinsky J.R., Welch G.R., Neimann H. 1997. Production of piglets preselected for sex following *in vitro* fertilization with X and Y chromosome–bearing spermatozoa sorted by flow cytometry. Ther., 47, 795-800.

Rath D., Johnson L.A., Welch G.R., Neimann H. 1994. Successful gamete intrafallopian tranfer (GIFT) in the porcine. Ther., 41, 1173-1179.

Rath D., Long C.R., Dobrinsky J.R., Welch G.R., Schreier L.L., Johnson L.A. 1999. *In vitro* production of sexed embryos for gender preselection: high speed sorting of X-chromosome-bearing sperm to produce pigs after embryo transfer J. Anim. Sci., 77, 3346-3352.

Renard J.P., Chastant S., Chesné P., Richard C., Marchal J., Cordonnier N., Chavatte P., Vignon X. 1999. Lymphoid hypoplasia and somatic cloning. The Lancet, 353, 1489-1491.

Reynolds J., Weir B.S., Cockerham C.C., 1983. Estimation of the coancestry coefficient: basis for a short-term genetic distance. Genetics, 105, 767-779.

Rinaldo D., Canope I., Christon R., 2000. The Créole pig of Guadeloupe: a review on reproduction, growth performance and meat quality in relation to dietary conditions. V Congreso iberoamericano de razas autòctonas y criollas, La Habana, 28 novembre-1er décembre 2000.

Robert A., Zamorano M.J., Ginés R., Argüello A., Delgado J.V. López J.L., 1998. Origen y estado actual del cerdo negro canario. II Congreso SERGA. Mallorca.

Rodero A., Delgado J.V., Rodero E., 1992. Primitive Andalusian livestock and their implications in the discovery of America. Arch. Zootec., 41, 383-400.

Rodero E., Delgado J.V., Camacho, M.E. Rodero A, 1994. "Conservación de razas andaluzas en peligro de extinción". Ediciones Junta de Andalucía. Sevilla.

Rohrer G.A., Alexander L.J., Hu Z., Smith T.P.L., Keele J.W., Beattie C.W., 1996. A comprehensive map of the porcine genome. Genome Res., 6, 371-391.

Rohrer G.A., Vögeli P. Stranzinger G., Alexander L.J., Beattie C.W., 1997. Mapping 28 erythrocyte antigen, plasma protein and enzyme polymorphisms using an efficient genomic scan of the porcine genome. Anim. Genet., 28, 323-330.

Ryder O.A., Benirschle K. 1997. The potential use of cloning in the conservation effort. Zoo. Biol., 16: 295-300.

Santiago E., Caballero A. 2000. Application of reproduction technologies to the conservation of genetic resources. Cons. Biol. (in press).

SAS, 1996. SAS/STAT software, release 6.12. SAS Institute Inc., Cary, NC.

Sather A.P., Jones S.D.M., Schaefer A.L., Colyn J., Robertson W.M., 1997. Feedlot performance, carcass composition and meat quality of free-range reared pigs. Can. J. Anim. Sci., 77, 225-232.

Scherf B., 2000. World Watch List for Domestic Animal Diversity 3rd edition. FAO, Rome.

Schön A., Brade W, 1996. Alte Schweinerassen im Test. In: Leistungsprüfungen in der Tierproduktion. LWK Hannover, 46-54. (s. also DLZ 3/97, 144-148).

Schröder H., 1997. Das Bunte Bentheimer Schwein. In: Gefährdete Schweinerassen. GEH/Hörning, 1997. NZH-Verlag Wetzlar. 41-46.

Schutz M.M., Freeman A.E., Lindberg G.L., Koehler C.M., Beitz D.C. 1994. The effect of mitochondrial DNA on milk production and health of dairy cattle. Liv. Prod. Sci., 72, 434-437.

Secondi F., Gandemer G., Bonneau M., Bernard E., Santucci P.P., Ecolan P., Casabianca F., 1996. Croissance, dévelopment tissulaire et caractéristiques de la carcasse du porc corse. Journées Rech. Porcine en France, 28, 109-114.

Serra X., Gil F., Pérez-Enciso M., Oliver M.A., Vàsquez J.M., Gispert M., Diaz I., Moreno F., Latorre R., Noguera J.L., 1998. A comparison of carcass, meat quality and histochemical characteristics of Iberian (Guadyerbas line) and Landrace pigs. Livest. Prod. Sci., 56, 215-223.

Setshwaelo L.L., 1990, Conservation of animal genetic resources in Africa. 4th World Congress Genet. Appl. Livest. Prod., 14, 449-454.

Shaw J.M., Oranratnachai A. and Trounson A.O. 2000. Fundamental cryobiology of mammalian oocytes and ovarian tissue. Ther., 53, 59-72.

Shiels P.G., Kind A.J., Campbell K.H.S., Waddington D., Wilmut I., Colman A., Schnieke A.E. 1999. Analysis of telomere lengths in cloned sheep. Nature, 399, 316-317.

Simon D.L., Buchenauer D., 1993. Genetic diversity of European livestock breeds EAAP publication n° 66, Wageningen Pers, Wageningen, The Netherlands.

Simon M.N., Segoviano V., Durand L., Liardou M.E., Juin H., Gandemer G., Legault C., 1996. Recherche de références sur les possibilités de valoriser les porcs Gascons et Limousins par le produits de qualité. 2. Qualités sensorielles de la viande. Journées Rech. Porcine en France, 28, 123-130.

Soong N.W., Hinton D.R., Cortopassi G., Arnheim N. 1992. Mosaicism for a specific somatic mitochondrial DNA mutation in adult human brain. Nat.Gen., 2, 318-329.

Steane D.E., 1991. Conservation of genetic resources in pigs and sheep. In Genetic Resources of Pig, Sheep and Goats (K. Maijala ed.), Elsevier, 145-155.

Suarez M.V., Barba C., Delgado J.V. Dieguez E., 1999. Comparative study of the reproductive performance of the Iberian pig varieties and Manchado de Jabugo. III Congreso SERGA and I Ibérico de conservación de recursos Genéticos. Lugo.

Suarez M.V., Barba C., Delgado J.V., Dieguez. E., 2001. Comparative study of the reproductive performance of the Iberian pig varieties and Manchado de Jabugo. Arch. Zootech. (in press).

Sun F.Z., Moor R. 1995. Nuclear transplantation in mammalian eggs and embryos. Curr. Top. Dev. Biol., 30, 147-176.

Sutherland R.A., Webb A.J., King J.W.B., 1985. A survey of world pig breeds and comparisons. Animal Breeding Abstracts, 53, 1-21.

Sztein J.M., O'Brien M.J., Farley J.S., Mobraaten L.E., Eppig J.J. 2000. Rescue of oocytes from antral follicles of crypreserved mouse ovaries: competence to undergo maturation, embryogenesis and development to term. Hum. Rep., 15, 567-571.

Takeda K., Takahashi S., Onishi A., Goto Y., Miyazawa A, Imai H. 1999. Dominant distribution of mitochondrial DNA from recipient oocytes in bovine embryos and offspring after nuclear transfer. J. Rep. Fert., 116, 253-259.

Telford N.A., Watson A.J., Schultz G.A. 1990. Transition from maternal to embryonic control in early mammalian development: a comparison of several species. Mol. Rep. Dev., 26, 90-100.

Thaon d'Arnoldi C., Foulley J.L., Ollivier L.,1998. An overview of the Weitzman approach to diversity. Genet. Sel. Evol., 30, 149-161.

Thilmant P. 1997. Congélation du sperme de verrat en paillette de 0.5 ml. Résultats sur le terrain. Ann. Méd. Vét., 141, 457-462.

Tonini G., 1953. La razza suina mora e i suoi derivati di incrocio, Stabilimento Grafico F. Lega, Faenza.

Toro M., Mäki-Tanila A. 1999. Establishing a conservation scheme. In "Genebanks and the conservation of farm animal genetic resources". J.K. Oldenbroek (ed.), 75-90. ID-DLO Institute for Animal Science and Health, Lelystad, The Netherlands.

Tucker M.J., Wright G., Morton P.C., Massey J.B. 1998. Birth after cryopreservation of immature oocytes with subsequent in vitro maturation. Fertil. Steril., 70), 578-579.

Vajta G., Holm P., Greve T., Callesen H. 1997. Vitrification of porcine embryos using Open Pulled Straw (OPS) method. Acta Vet. Scand., 38, 349-352.

Van der Wal P.G., Mateman G., de Vries A.W., Vonder G.M.A., Smulders F.J.M., Geesink G.H., Engel B., 1993. 'Scharrel' (free-range) pigs: carcass composition, meat quality and taste-panel studies. Meat Sci., 34, 27-37.

Van Zeveren A., Bouquet Y., Van de Weghe A., Coppieters W., 1990. A genetic blood marker study on 4 pig breeds. I-Estimation and comparison of within-breed variation. II-Genetic relationship between the populations. J. Anim. Breed. Genet., 107, 104-118.

Van Zeveren A., Peelman L., Van de Weghe A., Bouquet Y., 1995. A genetic study of four Belgian pig populations by means of seven microsatellite loci. J. Anim. Breed. Genet. 112, 191-204.

Wakayama T., Perry A.C.F., Zuccotti M., Johnson K.R., Yanagimachi R. 1998. Full-term development of mice from enucleated oocytes injected with cumulus cell nuclei. Nature, 394, 369-374.

Wakayama T., Rodriguez I., Perry A.C.F., Yanagimachi R., Mombaerts P. 1999. Mice cloned from embryonic stem cells. Proc. Nat. Acad. Sci. USA, 96, 14984-14989.

Wakayama T., Yanagimachi R. 1999. Cloning of male mice from adult tip cells. Nature Genetics, 22, 127-128.

Wallace D.C. 1992. Diseases of the mitochondrial DNA. An. Rev. Bioch., 61, 1175-1212.

Weitzman M. 1993. What to preserve? An application of diversity theory to crane conservation. Quarter. J. Econ., 108, 157-183.

Wells D.N., Misica P.M., Day A.M., Peterson A.J., Tervit H.R. 1998b. Cloning sheep from cultured embryonic cells. Rep. Fert. Dev., 10, 615-626.

Wells D.N., Misica P.M., Tervit H.R., Vivanco W.H. 1998a. Adult somatic nuclear transfer is used to preserve the last surviving cow of the Enderby Island cattle breed. Rep. Fertil. Dev., 10, 369-378.

Westendorf P., Richter L., Treu H., 1975. Zur Tiefgefrierung von Ebersperma. Labor-und Besamungsergebnisse mit dem Hulsenberger Pailleten-Verfahren. Dtsch. Tierärtz. Wsch., 82, 261-267.

White K.L., Bunch T.D., Mitalipov S., Reed W., 1999. Establishment of pregnancy after the transfer of nuclear transfer embryos produced from the fusion of Argali (Ovis ammon) nuclei into domestic sheep (Ovis aries) enucleated oocytes. Cloning, 1, 47-54.

Wildt D.E. 1992. Genetic resource banks for conserving wildlife species: justification, examples and becoming organized on a global basis. Anim. Rep. Sci., 28, 247-257.

Wilmut I., Schnieke A.E., McWhir J., Kind A.J., Campbell K.H.S. 1997. Viable offspring derived from fetal and adult mammalian cells. Nature, 385, 810-813.

Wood J.D., Jones R.C.D., Francombe M.A., Whelehan O.P., 1986. The effects of fat thickness and sex on pig meat quality with special reference to the problems associated with overleanness. 2 Laboratory and trained taste panel results. Anim. Prod., 43, 535-544.

Woolliams J.A., Wilmut I. 1999. New advances in cloning and their potential impact on genetic variation in livestock. Anim. Sci., 68, 245-256.

Yang X., Jiang S., Farrell P., Foote R.H., McGrath A.B. 1993. Nuclear transfer in cattle: effect of nuclear donor cells, cytoplasts age, co-culture, and embryo transfer. Mol. Rep. Dev., 35, 29-36.

Young L.E., Sinclair K.D. and Wilmut I. 1998. Large offspring syndrome in cattle and sheep. Rev. Rep., 3, 155-163.

Zakhartchenko V., Durcova-Hills G., Stojkovic M., Schernthaner W., Prelle K., Steinborn R., Muller M., Brem G., Wolf E. 1999. Effect of serum starvation and re-cloning on the efficiency of nuclear transfer using bovine fetal fibroblastst. J. Rep. Fert., 115, 325-331.

ZDS Jahresberichte 1990 - 1999. ADS/ZDS Bonn (Ed.).

Zetner K., 1969. Blutgruppen und biochemischer Polymorphismus bei Tuxer und Pustertaler Rindern. Dissertation Wien.

Zhang Z.G., 1986. Pig Breeds in China. Shanghai Scientific and Technical Publishers. Shanghai.

Zhao Z.L. 1990. The characteristics of Chinese pig breeds. In: Symposium sur le Porc Chinois (M. Molénat, C. Legault eds), 56-65, INRA Jouy en Josas.

Zheng Y.S., Fiser P., Sirad M.A. 1992. The use of ejaculated boar semen after freezing in 2 or 6% glycerol for in vitro fertilization of porcine oocytes matured in vitro. Ther., 38, 1065-1075.

Additional references on the Czech *Presticke* and Polish *Pulawska* breeds

Bzowska M., Karpowicz A., Ptak, J., Marciniak M., 2000. Pig Breeding Yearbook 1999. Central Animal Breeding Office, Warsaw, 72 pp.

Vachal J., 2000. Genetic Resources of Farm Animals in the Czech Republic. Ministry of Agriculture of the Czech Republic, Prague, 42 pp.